# MACRONUTRIENT

# BASICS

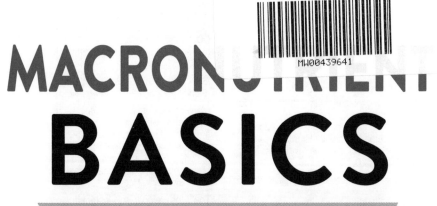

## INCLUDES 50+ RECIPES

## Your Guide to the Essentials of Macronutrients— and How a Macro Diet Can Work for You!

**MACRO GUIDELINES**

**STARTER RECIPES**

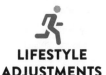

**LIFESTYLE ADJUSTMENTS**

MATT DUSTIN, CSCS

**Adams Media**
New York  London  Toronto  Sydney  New Delhi

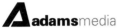 **adams**media

Adams Media
An Imprint of Simon & Schuster, Inc.
57 Littlefield Street
Avon, Massachusetts 02322

Copyright © 2020 by Simon & Schuster, Inc.

All rights reserved, including the right to reproduce this book or portions thereof in any form whatsoever. For information address Adams Media Subsidiary Rights Department, 1230 Avenue of the Americas, New York, NY 10020.

First Adams Media trade paperback edition January 2020

ADAMS MEDIA and colophon are trademarks of Simon & Schuster.

For information about special discounts for bulk purchases, please contact Simon & Schuster Special Sales at 1-866-506-1949 or business@simonandschuster.com.

The Simon & Schuster Speakers Bureau can bring authors to your live event. For more information or to book an event contact the Simon & Schuster Speakers Bureau at 1-866-248-3049 or visit our website at www.simonspeakers.com.

Interior images © Getty Images

Manufactured in the United States of America

10 9 8 7 6 5 4 3 2 1

Library of Congress Cataloging-in-Publication Data
Names: Dustin, Matt, author.
Title: Macronutrient basics / Matt Dustin, CSCS.
Description: Avon, Massachusetts: Adams Media, 2020.
Series: Basics.
Includes index.
Identifiers: LCCN 2019038550 | ISBN 9781507212707 (pb) | ISBN 9781507212714 (ebook)
Subjects: LCSH: Weight loss. | Carbohydrates. | Carbohydrates in human nutrition.
Classification: LCC RM222.2 .D788 2020 | DDC 613.2/83--dc23
LC record available at https://lccn.loc.gov/2019038550

ISBN 978-1-5072-1270-7
ISBN 978-1-5072-1271-4 (ebook)

Many of the designations used by manufacturers and sellers to distinguish their products are claimed as trademarks. Where those designations appear in this book and Simon & Schuster, Inc., was aware of a trademark claim, the designations have been printed with initial capital letters.

The information in this book should not be used for diagnosing or treating any health problem. Not all diet and exercise plans suit everyone. You should always consult a trained medical professional before starting a diet, taking any form of medication, or embarking on any fitness or weight training program. The author and publisher disclaim any liability arising directly or indirectly from the use of this book.

Always follow safety and commonsense cooking protocols while using kitchen utensils, operating ovens and stoves, and handling uncooked food. If children are assisting in the preparation of any recipe, they should always be supervised by an adult.

Contains material adapted from the following title published by Adams Media, an Imprint of Simon & Schuster, Inc.: *The Everything® Guide to Macronutrients* by Matt Dustin, CSCS, Pn1, copyright © 2017, ISBN 978-1-5072-0416-0.

# Contents

# Introduction

You may have heard of the health benefits of macronutrients—carbohydrates, fat, and protein. They're the source of the calories you consume and the building blocks of any diet, whether you're counting them to lose weight, boost energy, build lean muscle, or strengthen your heart. Each macronutrient serves a specific purpose, and you should consume it in the proper amount for the best health. But how can you plan your diet so you have the right balance of macronutrients?

Begin with the basics.

*Macronutrient Basics* teaches everything you need to know about macronutrients in a quick, easy-to-understand way. Wondering what macronutrients mean for your health? You'll find a systematic discussion of carbohydrates, fat, and protein and the role each should play in your eating habits. Want to know how many calories you should be eating? Here you'll find out the optimum number. Want to build the perfect diet plan? This book gives detailed advice about what to drink and eat. Plus, there are more than fifty delicious recipes that will help get your diet plan off to a good start!

In this book, you'll learn the ins and outs of macronutrients; how you apply this information is up to you. Maybe you're already on a diet but want to make some tweaks to it. Maybe you want to build lean muscle or increase your energy. Whatever your goal may be, this book will give you the tools to get there.

No matter what your reasons for learning more about macronutrients are, this book is here to help you confidently ease into this new lifestyle and apply it to your life—easily and effectively.

**1**

# Getting Started with Macronutrients

Macronutrients are the building blocks of any diet—proteins, carbohydrates, and fats—and they are where all of your calories come from (minus alcohol, which contains calories but is technically a toxin, so we don't count it as a macronutrient). Macronutrients supply the energy, fuel, and nutrients you need to live. Each macronutrient serves a specific purpose and should be consumed in the proper amount for optimal health. Quite a few variables come into play when setting up macronutrient ratios, but first, you must understand what they are, what they do, and what foods they come from.

# What Are Macronutrients?

Macronutrients form the basis of any nutrition plan. Regardless of whether you follow a strict diet plan or just eat whatever you feel like, you take in macronutrients every single day. Without an adequate macronutrient intake, your body would stop working. The amount of macronutrients in a given food determines how many calories are in that food. By figuring out exactly how many macronutrients your body needs each day and then eating that balanced amount, and adjusting your intake when things get stuck, you can achieve your health and weight loss goals.

# Carbs, Proteins, Fat

Macronutrients are carbs, proteins, and fat. An easy trick to remember this is remembering that macro means large. Micronutrients on the other hand, while essential, don't have any calories. Micronutrients would include vitamins, minerals, antioxidants, and other things found in food that don't have any calories.

# How Does Your Body Work?

To understand macronutrients, you need a very basic understanding of how your body operates. Every single process your body goes through every day, from brushing your teeth to digesting food and even breathing, requires energy. You may not feel physically tired from sitting on the couch watching television, but even the simple act of staying alive requires a little bit of energy. Your body gets the energy it needs from calories. Some foods have quite a few calories while some have very little, but all foods contain calories, even if they are found in very small amounts.

# What Do Calories Do?

A calorie is a measure of energy. In scientific terms, a calorie is the amount of energy needed to increase the temperature of 1 kilogram of water by 1°C. Thus, the more calories a food contains, the more energy it supplies to your body. A calorie isn't "good" or "bad"—it just is. Different foods will offer more nutritional benefits than others, but ultimately a calorie is still a calorie and nothing more than a measure of energy.

If you have a very active lifestyle, your body will use or "burn" a greater number of calories to function every day. Activities that make you feel physically tired, like running, playing sports, yard work, or significant walking, will burn more calories than sitting around doing nothing.

# Calories Are *Not* the Same As Fat

The human body is very smart. It can survive without food for weeks at a time under extreme circumstances, and it's a very complex operating system. Your body uses energy every single day, but it also stores excess energy for later use. Your body has a built-in system that allows it to save excess energy for a later time when you don't receive enough from food. This excess energy is stored in adipose cells, also known as body fat.

# Fats Are Essential for Life

That's right—that fat on your body contains stored energy, ready to be used when there isn't enough provided by the food you eat. Adipose tissue (body fat) provides some protection and insulation for your body, but at the end of the day, it's nothing more than stored energy. Eating more calories does not necessarily cause fat gain. If you're an athlete or work a physical job, you need to be eating extra calories just to function.

The problem lies in excess calorie consumption. If you regularly eat more calories than your body burns in a day, that excess energy needs to go somewhere, and most of it will be stored as body fat. If you eat fewer calories than your body needs, you'll end up using some of your stored fat for energy, decreasing your body fat stores. Body fat loss or gain ultimately comes down to calorie balance, and whether you're eating more than your body needs (fat gain), or less than your body needs (fat loss).

# Doesn't Fat Make You Fat?

No. This is a very common belief because they share the same name, but this is not true. Dietary fat that you eat in your food is essential for your body in certain amounts. Adipose tissue, or body fat, is simply stored calories. While eating foods high in fat can result in excess adipose tissue, consuming dietary fat in the correct amounts will not make you fat.

Dietary fat is simply another form of energy and nutrition; it does not directly correlate at all to actual body fat. The right fats supply the body with energy, help it retain crucial vitamins that require fat for absorption, protect the organs, and encourage healthy skin and hair.

# Create a Calorie Deficit

To lose fat, you must create a calorie deficit, which means you should eat fewer calories than your body burns in a day. A quick and easy way to create a caloric deficit is to stop drinking liquid calories. Soft drinks, fruit juices, fancy coffee drinks—all of these can be loaded with calories that don't fill you up whatsoever. Your first order of business should be removing calorie-containing drinks from your diet, except for the occasional alcoholic drink.

# Do You Need All Three Macronutrients?

As discussed, all calories come from macronutrients and alcohol, and each of these macros plays a unique role in how your body functions. If fat loss and body composition were a pyramid, total calories would form the base of that period, as that is the most important factor. However, the next level would be the actual quantities of macronutrients you consume each day.

# Balance Your Macronutrients

You must have a proper balance of the three macros. Having too much or too little of any of the three will lead to less than optimal health and body functioning, as all three play important roles, and none of them are bad or evil. You'll learn to figure out your exact macronutrient needs later in this book, as the required levels of each will vary based on your goals.

# Carbohydrates Are Fuel for Life

Carbohydrates, or carbs for short, come from starchy foods like potatoes, rice, and some other fruits and vegetables. They are the body's preferred source of energy for most activities, as they provide a quick form of easily accessible energy. Where protein and fats are slow to digest, and slow to break down to burn as fuel, carbohydrates are very easy for your body to digest, and stored carbohydrates are easy to use for energy. When you need a fast energy supply, carbohydrates will digest, absorb, and be used much more efficiently than protein or fats. Every gram of carbohydrate contains four calories. Technically, you could get by with no major health issues without including carbohydrates, as your body can create glucose from protein or fats, but it's very difficult to avoid carbohydrates entirely.

# Is Alcohol a Carbohydrate?

A gram of alcohol has seven calories, but as it doesn't provide any nutrition or any significant protein, carbohydrates, or fat, it's considered an "empty calorie." It gets you closer to your daily calorie goal without providing any value. If you consume alcohol and want to still hit your calorie goal for the day, you'll have to take away some calories from your daily food intake, and you'll lose that nutritional value. Often when tracking macros, it's suggested to take the alcohol calories from your carbohydrate and fat budget for the day if you choose to consume alcohol.

# The Role of Glycogen

Carbohydrates are broken down and stored throughout the body in the form of glycogen, mainly in the muscles and liver. Glycogen is a readily available fuel source for your body, particularly for high-intensity activities. If you're playing sports, exercising, or doing anything physically active, your body is most likely using stored glycogen to fuel those activities.

# Protein: Building Blocks

Proteins are made up of amino acids, which are the building blocks of most of the cells in the human body. Without amino acids, you'd be unable to replace the skin cells you lose every day, grow hair and fingernails, or rebuild and repair damaged muscle tissue. Proteins are essential for optimal health and body functioning. Every gram of protein has four calories. Protein comes from meat, fish, eggs, dairy products, and some lentils, such as soybeans. It's often consumed as a dietary supplement in powdered form, particularly among those who regularly exercise.

# Keeping Track: Calories or Macros?

When you're just getting started with a healthy eating plan, it may be enough to clean up your diet by eliminating soda, fast food, candy, and other foods that would typically be considered "bad."

This won't last forever. Eventually you're going to have to track and measure what you're eating, at least for a while. The closer you get to your goal weight, the harder it will be, and you'll really have to know exactly what's going in your body to continue making progress. With that being said, what should you be tracking? Calories or macros?

If you are tracking your macronutrients, you'll always know exactly how many calories you've consumed that day. It doesn't go both ways, however, as tracking calories alone can work for weight loss, but it isn't going to show you the exact macronutrient breakdown you're consuming, so you won't be able to optimize your health and performance the same way.

# The Importance of Food Labels

With food labels, it's very common for manufacturers to round up a bit just to make the label look a little cleaner. For example, if a food has 24 grams of protein, that would equate to 96 calories, but they may just round up to 100 calories for that food. If you're paying attention to your total macro intake and using some sort of app to track your food, don't worry if the calories are slightly off.

# The Basics of Food Tracking

If you're just getting started with food tracking, start by simply tracking total calories. This is easier to learn, and it'll build a good habit of paying attention to what you eat and what's in your food. Once you have this down, you can move on to tracking the specific macros you're consuming.

# Care about How You *Feel*

It's important to care about your internal health and how you feel, not just how you look. You can dramatically change your body composition and reduce fat by cutting your caloric intake down, but this doesn't mean you're healthy on the inside. Vitamins and minerals from whole, unprocessed food sources are essential to your immune system, hair and skin health, brain functioning, heart health, energy levels, and so many other important things.

# Macronutrients versus Micronutrients

You may be wondering, if macros are proteins, carbohydrates, and fats, where do are all of those vitamins and minerals come from? Surely those are important? The important nutritional value your food provides comes from micronutrients. These are the vitamins and minerals that allow your body to function at an optimal level. They are only required in small amounts, which is why they are called micronutrients, but they are very important. Your body is capable of hundreds of internal functions, with many of them happening simultaneously. Even something as simple as breathing requires the coordinated efforts of several different systems and muscles in your body.

# Go for Nutrient-Dense Foods

Nutrient-dense foods are the ones that provide the most nutritional value and should be a main staple of your diet. Foods like fruits, vegetables, lean proteins, whole grains, and healthy fats are all necessary to ensure you're getting the vitamins and minerals your body needs to run at 100 percent efficiency. Processed foods are often fortified with vitamins and minerals, but your best bet is to base your diet around whole foods.

# The Benefits of Nutrient-Dense Foods

While it's possible to change your body composition with any sort of food you'd like, assuming the calories add up, your overall health is far more important than the number on the scale. You may think you're cheating the system if you try to get all of your daily calories from foods that are lacking in micronutrients, but this isn't ideal if you care about your long-term health.

# Vitamin D

Vitamin D is the sunshine vitamin and is most commonly associated with mood and happiness. It's produced when your skin is exposed to sunlight on a regular basis, and a deficiency in vitamin D can lead to weak bones, depression, mood swings, rickets, cardiovascular problems, and many more issues. Although our bodies can produce vitamin D naturally, direct exposure to sunlight on a daily basis is required to initiate the natural production process, something many people don't get enough of. The best food sources for vitamin D are fatty fish, egg yolks, foods fortified with added vitamin D, or a supplement. If you are going to take a vitamin D supplement, be sure to check with your doctor first to figure out the right dosage for you as it's a fat-soluble vitamin that can accumulate in your system if you take more than your body can process.

# Vitamin C

Vitamin C is one that almost everybody knows as the immune system booster. When you start to get sick, you take extra vitamin C. While taking extra vitamin C when you're feeling under the weather can help strengthen your immune system, it's important to make sure you're getting enough even on the days when you aren't feeling sick. A lack of vitamin C has been linked to scurvy, a weak immune system, the tendency to bruise easily, and joint and muscle pain.

You can get vitamin C from oranges, kiwis, pineapple, papaya, kale, and various peppers. Eating a wide variety of fruits and vegetables every day is a good way to make sure you're getting plenty of this essential vitamin.

# Vitamin B

There are several different types of vitamin B, but they all do the same thing. These are water-soluble vitamins, which means they can be absorbed and utilized without relying on dietary fat. B vitamins help with cellular metabolism. They assist your body in absorbing the food you eat and using it for energy. These vitamins are also important for the formation of red blood cells, which transport oxygen to the various parts of your body.

You can supplement with vitamin B complexes, or you can obtain them from whole-food proteins like meat, fish, eggs, and leafy green vegetables.

# Vitamin K

Vitamin K is another fat-soluble vitamin that must be consumed with some dietary fat for your body to absorb it. Its most important role is in aiding with the formation of blood clots. If you cut yourself, you want your blood to form a clot as quickly as possible to stop the bleeding— a deficiency in vitamin K will make this very difficult. Foods high in vitamin K include spinach, asparagus, broccoli, lentils, eggs, and meats. If you're eating a well-rounded diet that includes a variety of fruits and vegetables, you're probably getting enough vitamin K. If you don't eat many vegetables, you might want to consider eating more or supplementing with vitamin K.

# Magnesium

Magnesium is a mineral found in dark leafy greens like spinach and kale, in addition to certain nuts. As researchers are learning more about this mineral, it's becoming quite clear that it's one of the most important minerals you can consume, and magnesium deficiency is becoming a dangerous epidemic.

Most leafy greens used to be very high in magnesium, but as modern farming methods have changed, the nutritional content of plants has started to decline. Magnesium deficiency can cause muscle cramping, muscle spasms, hormonal issues, high blood pressure, mood swings and depression, anxiety, lack of energy, and problems sleeping. It's extremely important to consume optimal levels of magnesium, and unless you are eating a lot of leafy greens every day, a supplement may be beneficial as a nutritional insurance.

# Potassium

Potassium is an electrolyte, which is a mineral that helps your body send signals through the muscles. Without adequate potassium, your body's nerves may not function properly, and you may experience muscle cramping or twitching and have difficulty contracting your muscles the proper way. Because your body loses electrolytes when you sweat, it's important to get plenty of potassium in your diet if you lead an active life. It is possible to have too much potassium, but a healthy liver will remove any excess potassium from your blood. Eating potassium-rich foods like bananas, spinach, squash, and avocados is the best way to ensure you are getting enough from natural food sources. If you tend to sweat a lot and notice muscle cramps during exercise, you may want to consume an electrolyte drink during your workouts to stay hydrated.

# Calcium

Of all the minerals found in your body, calcium is the one you have in the greatest abundance, and up to 99 percent of it is stored in your bones and teeth. Beyond supporting a strong skeletal system, calcium also plays an important role in blood vessel and muscular contractions, as well as in the production of certain hormones and enzymes.

Calcium is primarily found in dairy products, so including milk, yogurt, and cheese in your diet is a good way to make sure you're getting enough calcium. It's also found in some dark leafy greens and can be supplemented if you follow a vegan diet that doesn't allow any dairy product intake.

# 2

# Understanding Macronutrients

Just as all foods are not created equal, all macros are not created equal. This chapter will give you an in-depth look at proteins, carbohydrates, and fats, showing you what your best choices are in each macronutrient category. This chapter will also debunk a few common macronutrient myths and illuminate how some other restrictive diets can actually hurt your body while flexible eating allows you to keep your systems in proper working order. Having a better understanding of each macronutrient will allow you to make the best choices for your health and diet goals.

# Simple versus Complex Carbs

You've probably heard of simple carbs and complex carbs. This simply refers to the speed at which they are broken down, digested, and absorbed into your bloodstream. Simple carbs are fast-digesting and complex carbs are slow-digesting. Cereal, sugary snacks, rice, and fruit would be considered simple carbs, while foods like leafy green vegetables, whole grains, oats, and high-fiber carb sources would be considered more complex.

Carbohydrates often contain fiber. Fiber is very important for heart health, digestion, and controlling blood sugar. Foods that are higher in fiber will take longer to digest and will generally keep you full longer. The exact ranges vary from person to person based on factors like age, gender, and weight, but most people should aim to consume 25–40 grams of fiber per day.

# The Glycemic Index

Digestion speed is measured by something called the glycemic index. High-glycemic carbs are the ones that digest quickly and low-glycemic carbs digest a bit more slowly.

High-glycemic carbs come from foods like fruit, rice, candy, soda, juice, and any other "sugary" carb. They digest quickly and give you a quick hit of energy. Low-glycemic carbs come from whole grains, vegetables, and any carbohydrate that's a bit slow to digest. These typically take longer to break down, so you'll feel full longer and have a steady, slow release of energy.

# Are There "Bad Carbs"?

Typically when someone talks about "bad carbs," they are referring to sugary, processed carb sources. These are things like candy, soda, fruit juice, or just about anything else that's sweet, delicious, and comes from a box, and often people like to blame sugar for their problems. The truth is, all carbohydrates are made up of simple sugar molecules.

When fully broken down by your body's digestive system, carbohydrates are made up of either glucose or fructose, two simple sugar molecules. It doesn't matter if you get 40 grams of carbs from cake or from brown rice; those 40 grams of carbs will eventually end up as simple glucose molecules, the same as sugar.

# Get Carbs from Whole Foods

In terms of pure body composition, the carb source doesn't really matter. It's important to know this so that you don't associate desserts, soda, or any other carbs you enjoy with guilt and immediate fat gain. For optimal health, you should be getting most of your carbs from whole foods. However, the occasional treat, assuming it fits into your daily calorie allotment, isn't going to derail your progress. It's much better to allow yourself to enjoy these treats in moderation if it helps you stay on track, rather than attempt to eliminate them completely and end up caving in and eating a whole cake on the weekend.

# Sources of Carbs

To help you plan your diet, here is a list of whole foods that contain primarily carbohydrates. Some foods will contain high amounts of multiple macronutrients, but these foods are mostly carbs. There will be similar lists for proteins and fats as well. The best way to learn which macros are in which foods is to start checking the nutritional information labels of the foods you buy, but the following lists will give you a quick reference guide to look at.

## Carbohydrate Sources

- Bread
- Fruit
- Oatmeal
- Pasta
- Potatoes
- Rice
- Squash

# The Varieties of Protein

Just like carbohydrates are classified as simple or complex, proteins also come in two varieties: complete and incomplete. Remember how proteins are made up of amino acids? Well, of those amino acids, nine are referred to as essential amino acids. Essential amino acids cannot be produced by the human body and must be obtained through food or supplements.

Protein is what allows you to rebuild your body and recover from the daily wear and tear you place on it. Often people associate high protein intake with gaining muscle, but that's just one role protein plays in the body. Every day, your body is regenerating hair, skin, fingernails, and yes, muscle tissue. It uses amino acids to do this, so if you aren't consuming enough from your diet, your body will start to rip apart and break down your muscle tissue to get those amino acids.

# The Thermic Effect

In terms of digestion, there is something called the thermic effect of food. Remember how every process in your body requires energy? Digestion is no different. Every food you eat requires some energy to break it down, absorb it, and put it to use or store for later. Protein has a high thermic effect, which means it burns quite a few calories simply from digesting it—roughly 20–30 percent of the calories in a solid protein will be burned from digesting it, and that number is closer to 5–10 percent for most carbs and fats. You shouldn't try to adjust the total calorie content based on this, but it's good to know. The more solid proteins you eat, the more calories you'll burn simply from digestion.

# Complete and Incomplete Proteins

If a protein source contains all nine essential amino acids, it's considered a complete protein. If it's lacking any of the essential amino acids, it's considered an incomplete protein. It's important that you get plenty of complete proteins throughout the day, whatever your diet of choice may be. It's possible to supplement with amino acids, and many companies produce "branched-chain" or essential amino acid supplements. It's still better to get these amino acids from whole-food sources, but if you find you are struggling to get enough protein in your diet, an inexpensive essential amino acid supplement could help.

# Vegans: Why You Still Need Proteins

If you're a vegan or vegetarian, you still need complete proteins if you want to live a healthy life. Unfortunately, most plant-based proteins just aren't complete. Soy protein is one of the few complete plant proteins available, but excess soy consumption can have negative side effects, so try not to go overboard with the soy protein. If you follow a vegan diet, especially if you are active, you should strongly consider investing in a plant-based protein supplement to ensure you are reaching your daily goals, and get a wide variety of protein sources to get your essential amino acids.

# Growing New Muscle

What actually causes you to grow new muscle?

While protein plays a role in muscle growth, it's only a small part of the picture. Muscle growth, or hypertrophy, is the combined result of heavy resistance training that's performed consistently over a long period of time and excess caloric intake. If you're eating more than you need, getting adequate protein, and training your muscles with the appropriate intensity, you'll slowly start to gain more muscle. It doesn't happen simply from increasing your protein intake, so you won't accidentally get too big or anything.

# The Myth of Proteins and Kidney Damage

You may have heard that eating too much protein or using protein supplements will damage your kidneys. This simply isn't true. Your body has to work harder to break down protein, but if anything, this is a good thing. Even at doses as high as 2 grams per pound of body weight (which is far more than anyone needs), protein intake is very safe.

# Sources of Protein

Here are some important sources of protein for you to work into your diet.

## Protein Sources

- Beef
- Chicken
- Dairy products
- Eggs
- Fish
- Protein powder
- Turkey

# Good Fats and Bad Fats

In terms of dietary fat, there are several different kinds. The exact science of how they are classified is not necessary to know; just know that unsaturated fats are the best, saturated fats are decent, and trans fats should be avoided whenever possible. You also have monounsaturated fats and polyunsaturated fats, but the easiest thing is just to remember which foods provide the "good" fats.

# The Benefits of Healthy Fats

Contrary to common belief, fat is not evil. The word itself sounds bad because it's often associated with body fat, which many people want to lose. The truth is, you need dietary fat for your body to function. There are good fats and bad fats, and some are better than others, but without adequate fat intake, you'll run into all sorts of health problems.

# Saturated and Unsaturated Fats

Avoid trans fats whenever possible. There are a few different types of fats, classified based on their molecular structure. They are unsaturated fats, saturated fats, and trans fats. Generally speaking, unsaturated fats and some saturated fats, which are found in avocados, egg yolks, red meat, nuts, coconut, and fish, are the "good fats." Trans fats, on the other hand, have been associated with a higher risk of heart disease and other negative effects. They are often found in fried and heavily processed foods.

# Dietary Fat and Hormones

The last important function of dietary fat is hormonal support. Fat supplies cholesterol, which is generally classified as HDL or LDL cholesterol. Too much cholesterol, particularly too much LDL cholesterol, can cause plaque formation and buildup in your heart. However, not getting enough cholesterol is also bad.

Cholesterol is important for producing many hormones in the body, including important reproductive hormones, which is why those who follow very low-fat diets often report negative hormonal changes after a while. There's no need to go overboard with fat, but don't be afraid of including the right fats in your diet.

# Omega-3s

The best sort of fat you can get is one that's high in omega-3 fatty acids. There are two common omegas: omega-3 fatty acids and omega-6 fatty acids. Omega-3s are found in fatty cuts of fish, egg yolks, avocados, and nuts, as well as a few other foods, and they can also be supplemented. Foods that are high in omega-3s are considered to be good fats.

# Omega-6s

Omega-6 fatty acids are very common in processed and fried foods like salad dressings, pizza, French fries, and sausages, in addition to certain cooking oils, such as vegetable oil. Omega-6 fatty acids are a tricky subject. They are essential, in that your body needs them and cannot produce them, but it's important to have the right balance between omega-6 and omega-3 fatty acids.

# Sources of Fat

It's very common to have a diet that's much higher in omega-6s, as people tend to eat a lot of processed vending machine snacks and fast food. If your omega-6 fatty acid intake outweighs your omega-3 intake, you'll run into health problems, like increased inflammation and increased risk of cardiovascular disease. To get as close to a one-to-one ratio of omega-6 and omega-3 fatty acids as possible, be sure to eat plenty of good fats on a regular basis, and minimize processed and fried food intake.

## Fat Sources

- Avocado
- Coconut oil
- Cooking oils such as olive oil and macadamia nut oil
- Egg yolks
- Fatty cuts of fish
- Nuts
- Red meat

# Balance Macronutrients for Health

A healthy diet will consist of a balance of all three macronutrients. The most commonly recommended ratio is 40 percent protein, 40 percent carbohydrates, and 20 percent fat. Later chapters will detail exactly how to calculate your exact ratios based on your goals and lifestyle factors, but these numbers are a good general recommendation. The total number of calories in your diet are determined by your macronutrient intake. If you decrease your total calorie intake, all of your macronutrient numbers will decrease as well. For a healthy, safe approach to weight loss, you should keep a balance of all three nutrients in your diet, rather than eliminating one altogether.

# Low-Carb Diets

One of the most common diets is the low-carb or even zero-carb diet. While protein and fats are essential to live and be healthy, carbohydrates are not, so if a low-carb diet was followed correctly, it wouldn't have any serious health consequences. However, for most people, it just isn't realistic to give up carbs completely for any long period of time. You'll have to eat extra fats to make up for those lost calories, and unless you're careful, it's easy to eat too much of the wrong sorts of fats and end up with health issues down the road. You may also find yourself short on a lot of micronutrients if you limit things like fruits and vegetables.

Unless you are following a carb-cycling diet, which is not necessary and is a bit more advanced, it's probably best to avoid low-carb diets. It's not an unhealthy option and in theory it makes sense. However, giving up carbohydrates for good just isn't realistic for most people, and it would be more beneficial to learn to follow a balanced diet. The best diet is the one you can sustain for a long time.

# Losing Water Weight

For every gram of glycogen your body stores, it also stores 3 grams of water. This means that if you remove carbohydrates from your diet completely, you'll drop a lot of water weight from your muscle and liver cells. Don't confuse this for fat loss if you follow a low-carb diet; that initial weight drop is mostly water. This works both ways; if you eat a high-carbohydrate meal, you'll hold excess water. No need to panic if the scale jumps overnight after a carb-heavy meal.

# Low-Fat Diets

This type of diet is the one with the most potential to do more harm than good. Many people used to think that dietary fat was what caused fat gain, which remains a common misconception. You know the truth now, that excess calories are to blame and fats are okay.

When your fat intake drops too low, your hormonal levels will suffer. Hormones, particularly reproductive hormones, are dependent on fat. For both men and women, removing too much fat from a diet can lead to decreased energy, mood swings, and a decreased sex drive. Women often report irregular menstrual cycles as well when dietary fat intake drops too low.

Even if weight loss is your primary goal, you should still be concerned with your overall health first and foremost. Cutting out fat may help you lose weight, but it's probably going to have some serious negative side effects.

# Ketogenic Diets

The ketogenic diet is one of the most popular diets right now, with keto books, blogs, recipes, and supplements popping up everywhere. The goal of a true ketogenic diet is to keep carbohydrate intake very low, with a moderate protein intake and a high dietary fat intake. This is different from what most people would consider keto: simply removing carbs while keeping protein high. There is some interesting research being done on the possible health benefits of the ketogenic diet in medical situations, including potential anticancer benefits, but for now it's too early to say definitely if the ketogenic diet should be used in medical settings.

# The Problem with the Ketogenic Diet

There is nothing bad about the ketogenic diet, but there's nothing magical either. It doesn't change the rules of thermodynamics or human physiology; to lose fat you must be in a calorie deficit, keto or not. Some people see tremendous results following the ketogenic diet, but it's also very common for people to gain weight when starting.

Remember that fat has 9 calories, compared to the 4 calories in protein and carbs. By removing carbohydrates and drastically increasing your fat intake, it's very easy to significantly increase your calorie intake and begin to store body fat. It can also be tough to keep the proper balance of fats; if you start adding bacon and butter to your meals, you might run into long-term health issues with your cholesterol. Finally, if you're into any sort of athletics or performance, the ketogenic diet is not optimal for performance. You'll be able to finish your workouts just fine, but you'll never perform as well as you would with carbohydrates.

# Who Should Use a Ketogenic Diet?

While a low-carb diet is useful for a lot of people, the actual ketogenic diet, which is also pretty low protein and very high fat, is difficult to stick with. Your body eventually adapts to running on fats, but taking in any carbohydrates resets the system, and you have to go through the adaptation process all over again, which is not pleasant, and often referred to as keto flu. The ketogenic diet would be a good fit for anyone who's willing to put a lot of time into tracking and planning, to make sure they have the right balance of fats, as well as someone willing to give up carbohydrates indefinitely. It would also work well for someone who's not very physically active. For anyone else, the diet will be extremely difficult to follow for any significant length of time.

# Make Healthy Choices

In a perfect world, all of your food would come from fresh, whole-food sources and supply perfectly balanced nutrition. In the real world, this simply isn't realistic for most people. Life is meant to be enjoyed, and you shouldn't have to make yourself miserable or become obsessed with your food choices to be healthy and maintain the body you want.

If you can learn to fit those indulgences into your daily macronutrients without losing control and binge eating an entire pizza in one sitting, you'll find you can enjoy the foods you love on a regular basis and still see fantastic results. A very good rule of thumb is the 80/20 rule: 80 percent of your food should be from whole, unprocessed foods sources, while up to 20 percent can be from the more processed foods.

# Know Your Goals

In order to build your perfect diet plan, you must first decide what your goals are. Are you looking to just lose weight? Are you looking to gain more muscle? Your final goal will influence your eating plan and how many macros you will require each day. Once you have your goals in mind, the next chapter will show you how to calculate the proper amount of calories and macronutrients that you should be eating each day. With your macronutrient amounts calculated, you can then create your eating plan, including what times you should eat and what your meals should consist of. Proper planning is key to success on the macronutrient diet.

## 3

# The Macronutrient Diet Is Your Friend

There are many different diet plans available, and with so many to choose from, it's important to choose the one that's a good fit for your individual lifestyle and preferences. The macronutrient diet is easily adaptable to any dietary schedule, lifestyle, and preference. This chapter will take you through both the science of the macronutrient diet and also the wide range of benefits that this flexible diet offers. You'll also learn about your body's different energy-burning cycles and how properly integrating your macronutrients throughout the day can help your progress.

# Adjust Your Diet to Your Goal

As you assemble your meal plan, consider your primary goal. Is it body composition and the number on the scale or performing your best during your workouts or athletic activities? For pure body composition, meal timing doesn't matter at all. As long as your numbers add up at the end of the day, you'll be just fine. If you are trying to lose weight without exercising and focus only on your nutrition, you can set up your meal plan however you'd like without worrying about meal timing.

# Weight Loss versus Muscle Gain

Whether your goal is to lose weight or build some muscle, you'll need to adjust your current calorie intake. Remember that losing fat requires a caloric deficit, or eating less than you burn in a day. The opposite is true for building muscle—you need to eat more than you need and give your body the extra food it needs to grow. In general, you can be a bit more aggressive when trying to lose fat than when trying to gain muscle. While it is possible to lose weight too quickly, it's much more preferable to lose weight fast and adjust to slow it down. You'll just look better faster, which can build some momentum and motivation.

# Body Composition

Body composition simply refers to the ratio of fat to lean tissue you carry. A higher body fat percentage means that more of your total body weight comes from fat, as opposed to lean tissue, bones, and organs. When someone mentions improving body composition, they are generally referring to reducing body fat while maintaining, or even building, lean muscle tissue. Improving body composition is the fastest way to visually look better and get other people noticing that your body is changing.

As far as body composition is concerned, flexible dieting is the most precise way to control your food intake and make small adjustments as needed. If you always have an idea of exactly where your calories are at, as well as your individual macronutrients, it's easy to make a small adjustment, like removing 30 grams of carbs from your daily intake, or adding 10 grams of fat, things like that. An untracked diet makes it impossible to be precise, and this precision is needed to push through plateaus and continue to see results.

# Take a Controlled Approach to Muscle Building

With muscle building, you should take a slow, controlled approach. Start with only small increases, see how your body responds, and increase again as needed. A common mistake is for people to start eating everything in sight when they want to build muscle and then end up gaining more body fat than they intended. When building muscle, the goal is to build actual muscle—not simply make the scale move up by gaining fat as well.

# Eating and Exercise

If you're an active person and want to perform your best and recover from your exercise, meal timing comes into play a bit more. Carbohydrates play a large role in both fueling your exercise and helping you recover. It makes sense then to place a significant portion of your carbohydrates before and after intense physical activity, as this will give you the most benefit from them. This is especially important if you're dieting, and your carbohydrates are getting lower and lower.

# How to Find Your Exact Numbers

It's time to get into the actual numbers. You'll start by figuring out your maintenance calorie intake, which is roughly how many calories your body uses every day. To lose fat, you'll eat fewer calories than your maintenance levels, and to build muscle, you'll eat above maintenance.

There are many ways to do this, and none will ever be 100 percent accurate. So, to figure out your fat loss calories, which you'll need to track and adjust as you go, you'll need a bit of trial and error in the beginning. Keep in mind that so many factors affect your caloric output—activity levels, genetics, body composition, nutrition, and many more. The math you're about to do will be a best guess, so don't expect to get your calories perfect on the first try. You'll want to set up your initial numbers, track for a week or two, then assess. That is the only way to know if you're on track; if you aren't, you need to adjust.

# Men and Women and Calories

Why do women need fewer calories than men? Women naturally have lower levels of muscle than men do. They don't have quite as much testosterone and growth hormone, either, so building muscle is a bit more challenging. Because muscle tissue burns calories even at rest, the higher levels of muscle in men, along with higher levels of testosterone and growth hormone, mean that men typically burn more calories per pound than women do. Women also tend to weigh less, so daily activities will burn fewer calories.

# Step One: Figure Out Your Total Calories

If you're a man, multiply your body weight by 14. If you're a woman, multiply your body weight by 12. This will give you a rough guess at your total calories needed to maintain your body weight. Now that you've come up with a number for your calories, the next step is to consume calories according to this number as closely as you can for seven to ten days. Check your body weight on day one and day ten to compare.

If you lose weight, you've found a caloric deficit. If fat loss is your goal, this is perfect. If you lost more than two and a half pounds, however, that's too fast, and you're undereating. You'll want to bump food up a bit. If you gained weight, you're eating above maintenance. Lower your food intake by a few hundred calories and try again. You want to start with a 15 percent decrease in calories, eat that number for a few days, and then check your weight again, repeating until you find your maintenance level.

If your weight stayed the same, you found your maintenance intake. To lose fat, take about 500 calories away from your total carbs and fats. If you want to add muscle, add about 300 calories primarily to carbs with some going to fat.

# Step Two: Calculate Your Macros

Now that you have your total calories, it's time to split those calories up into their respective macros. Remember, protein and carbohydrates each have 4 calories per gram, while fat has 9 calories per gram. If you want to plan to include alcohol, it has 7 calories per gram but zero nutritional value, so you'll have to lower your remaining calories and simply eat less carbs and fat.

- **Protein:** Set your protein at 1 gram per pound of lean body weight, which is different from total body weight (refer to the formula in this chapter for Lean Body Mass Calculation). Write that number down.
- **Fat:** Now set your fat anywhere between 0.25–0.45 grams per pound (lower if you prefer higher carbs, and vice versa).
- **Carbs:** Your remaining calories, after protein and fat, will go to carbs. On training days, set your carbs at 1.25–1.5 grams per pound of body weight, depending on how you ended up setting your fat (higher or lower). On rest days, set your carbs at 0.5 grams per pound and increase fat by 0.10 grams per pound.

# Macro to Calorie Conversions

The math here may seem complicated, but follow along if you can with your own bodyweight. This example will use a 200-pound male with roughly 15 percent body fat, looking to lose fat. For total calories, use 14 times total body weight for men, so for the sample calculations, total maintenance calories will be 2,800.

For fat loss, it's best to start with a 500-calorie per day deficit. Therefore, our fictional man's total calorie intake goals will be 2,300 calories per day. For the rest of the calculations, use the following conversion chart.

## Macro to Calorie Conversions

- 1 gram protein = 4 calories
- 1 gram carbohydrate = 4 calories
- 1 gram fat = 9 calories

# Lean Body Mass Calculation

Use the following equations to determine various body mass calculations for yourself.

1.  Total body weight × body fat percentage = pounds of fat.

2.  Total body weight − pounds of fat = lean body mass. Remember, the sample person weighs 200 pounds at 15 percent body fat.

3.  200 × 0.15 (15 percent) = 30 pounds of fat.

4.  200 pounds − 30 pounds = 170 pounds lean body mass.

# Protein Calculations

Protein should be set at 1 gram per pound of lean body weight. At 170 pounds of lean body mass, this means protein will be set at 170 grams every day.

Protein calories are 170 × 4, or 680.

# Fat Calculations

Fat should be set at 0.25–0.45 grams per pound of body weight. Since the man weighs 200 pounds and prefers higher-fat meals, he'll use 0.45 grams:

>200 pounds × 0.45 grams means fat will be set at 90 grams per day. Fat calories are 90 × 9, or 810.

# Carb Calculations

To calculate carbohydrates, take your protein and fat calories and subtract them from your total calories for the day. The remaining calories are used for carbohydrates.

Total calories – protein calories – fat calories = carbohydrate calories. 2,300 – 680 – 810 = 810 carbohydrate calories.

Now that you have 810 carbohydrate calories, simply divide this number by 4 to figure out how many grams of carbohydrates are to be consumed each day:

810 divided by 4 = 203 grams of carbohydrates every day.

# Total Calorie Calculations

Therefore, the final goal numbers for each day are 2,300 calories, coming from 170 grams of protein, 90 grams of fat, and 203 grams of carbohydrates. Use these calculations to figure out your individual daily needs for total calories and total macros, and use those numbers to plan your days and meal plans. In general, you don't need to hit every macro to the exact gram every day, they are just targets. If you can get all macros within 5–10 grams over/under for your macros consistently, you should be able to see good results without stressing accuracy too much.

# Build Your Perfect Meal Plan

There's a famous quote about planning that states, "Failing to plan is planning to fail," and when it comes to dietary adherence, this is 100 percent true. If you aren't planning your nutrition ahead of time, there's no way you can have any shot at consistently hitting your macros for any long period of time. Guessing, hoping it works out, and adjusting on the fly is stressful and time-consuming. Rather than take a reactive approach to your diet and adjust as you go, be proactive and plan your days ahead of time. This way, before the day even starts, you'll see exactly what your macro intake will look like, and you can plan ahead to fill any gaps, or adjust as needed.

If you prefer a more rigid schedule and less planning stress, try planning out two or three perfect days that hit your macros dead-on, and then just follow those meal plans. When coming up with your plans, make sure at least 80 percent of your diet consists of unprocessed whole foods, and make sure your plans are realistic.

# Step One: Figure Out Your Schedule

Start by looking at an average day in your life. How many meals can you eat? When are you the busiest? When do you have the most time to cook? If you work from home, chances are you'll have an easier time preparing three to four meals per day. If you're a busy executive who's constantly working long days and rushing in and out of meetings, you may find that you need a quick and easy breakfast, a few snacks, and a big dinner.

Regardless of your schedule, figure out what sort of meal plan would be easy for you to follow in terms of timing and write those meals down, times and all.

# Step Two: Divide Your Macros

Now that you have your meal times, and total number of meals, attempt to evenly split your macros across each meal. If your goal is 140 grams of protein per day, and you eat four meals, you'd want to aim for around 35 grams with each meal. This makes hitting your macros much more manageable, rather than trying to get all of your protein at once.

If you're working out that day, put most of your carbs before and after your workout, otherwise you can spread them around however you'd like. For each meal, write down the total number of macronutrients and calories you'll need for that meal.

# Step Three: Choose Your Foods

Now you have the framework and basic structure of how your day will look, and it's time to fill it in. Look at each meal and figure out what foods will give you that meal's required calories and macros. This is where you can have fun and get really creative. The recipes in this book include nutrition calculations that will tell you exactly how many macros are in each serving. This makes planning easy, though of course you can use any food you like.

# Keep Macros Around the House

If you don't want to follow premade recipes, a simple trick is to pick three carbs, three proteins, and two to three high-fat foods to keep around your house at all times. This way, you can mix and match ingredients to plan your meals as needed. Most foods will have the nutritional information right on the package. For produce, nearly all fruits are higher in carbohydrates, while green vegetables will have fewer carbohydrates. For your carbs, you can choose fruit, rice, oats, and potatoes, for example, with your proteins coming from meats, eggs, and maybe protein powder. You can choose different combinations of foods, adding fat as needed through things like cooking oils and butter, or choosing higher-fat cuts of meat, like red meat or fatty fish.

# Choose High-Fiber Macros

When choosing food sources, keep in mind that foods high in fiber will keep you full the longest, making it easier to diet. Choose leafy greens, whole grains, and assorted fruits and vegetables to fight off hunger during the day.

If you're making a recipe or meal that doesn't have the calculated macros, simply add up all the ingredients you're using, divide by the number of servings the meal provides, and use those numbers as your macronutrient intake for the meal.

# There's an App for That

By the end of all this planning, you should have a sample meal plan that fits your schedule perfectly, allows you to hit your macros, and uses foods of your choosing—not random foods from a magazine meal plan. You can write out the foods you want by hand, or use an app for a food log, like MyFitnessPal, Cronometer, or Mike's Macros. This way you can plan the next day ahead of time and see where any gaps may be that you need to fill. Planning, and sticking to the plan, sets you up for the best possible chance at success as it's a plan perfectly engineered for your needs, schedule, and preferences.

# Adjust Your Numbers

While something like trying to lose a bit of belly fat may not seem like the end of the world, your body simply sees a diet as a period of restricted food, and it will act accordingly. Typically, a few weeks of reduced food intake will trigger your body to learn to function at its new calorie level, and any weight loss will slow down. Not to mention, if you lose fat and weigh less, you'll be burning fewer calories just from your normal daily activities.

When these situations pop up, it's important to understand how to adjust your diet so that you can continue to make progress toward your goal. If you want to increase that energy deficit so you continue to burn fat, you can either reduce your food intake or work to burn more calories.

# Diet and Metabolism

While it's true that your body's metabolism will slow down the longer you diet, it's not necessarily true metabolic damage. After all, both your body weight and food intake will be lowered, so it makes sense that your metabolism will slow down. Unless you have a history of eating disorders or have dieted down to dangerously low levels multiple times, you probably don't have real metabolic damage—you just need to lower your calories, as your body has adapted.

This could be due to several reasons. Most likely, your body's metabolism has simply adjusted, and because you now weigh less, you don't need as much food, so weight loss will slow down. You may also see a slight decrease in the production of hormones that regulate fat loss, such as the thyroid hormones. In more extreme cases of prolonged, severe caloric restriction, it's possible that your body will actually fight weight loss because it thinks that it's not getting enough food, so it wants to hang on to the energy stores it has, but this is rare, and most of the time it's normal metabolic adaptation, not a health issue.

# When to Adjust

For both weight loss and weight gain, dieting is rarely a linear process. Over the course of a week, it's very common for your body weight to fluctuate on a daily basis. Hormonal issues, sodium intake, hydration levels, food that's still being processed through your digestion and waste system…all of these factors can increase or decrease the number you see on your scale. It's best to weigh yourself only once per week at the most. Pick a day and time that you know will be consistent. Some people prefer Monday weigh-ins, although you may be a bit heavier if you ate foods over the weekend that aren't normally part of your diet. Others prefer midweek or Friday weigh-ins, as this lets your body settle into a normal routine, allowing for a more accurate reading. The most accurate option is to weigh yourself every day, and track your weekly average, though the daily weigh-in can be stressful for some.

# How to Adjust

Start by adjusting your carbohydrates first. As these are the only non-essential macronutrient, most adjustments should come from carbohydrates. Whether your goal is fat loss or muscle gain, the simplest method is to set protein and fat at optimal levels for health and performance and then simply manipulate your carbohydrate intake up or down, based on your goal. Start with a 10 percent total calorie adjustment. If you've been dieting at 2,000 calories and you've been stuck for two weeks, adjust your calories down to 1,800. This may not be aggressive enough, but it's always better to go slowly and take your time rather than slash your food intake too low, too quickly. If your carbs start to get low, you can also lower fats slightly as well, though they should never drop below 40 grams.

# Simple Carbs Are Best for Workouts

Fast-digesting carbohydrates give you both the fuel you need to perform and the materials you need to recover and rebuild. Placing carbohydrates before and after your workouts is the easiest way to make sure you can work hard and recover as fast as possible.

When it comes to workouts, simple carbohydrates are best. Fruits, rice, bread, or sports drinks are excellent options. Avoid foods that contain too much fiber or fat, as both of these can slow down digestion, because your priority is digesting those carbs so that your body can use them. While high-fiber carbs like oatmeal or leafy vegetables are fine, they may not be optimal for immediately before and after workouts.

# Eat Guilt-Free

Not only can an unplanned indulgence send you way over your daily or even weekly calories; it is also the most common cause of dietary guilt. If you've been tracking your macros consistently and suddenly you get thrown way off track by a cheat meal, it can make you feel like a failure, and it'll be hard to get back on track. This is dangerous for long-term success.

# Plan Ahead

The trick to eating foods you enjoy is planning ahead. If you know that tomorrow night is pizza night, open up tomorrow's food log, plug in however much pizza you want to eat, and adjust the rest of your day accordingly. Being proactive about this will allow you to go through your day stress-free, knowing you'll hit your targets even with that added pizza, and you can enjoy your treat without feeling bad.

## 4

# Benefits, Risks, and Concerns of the Macronutrient Diet

Now that you have a big-picture understanding of how nutrition works, it's time to look at how to eat for maximum health. While calories are the biggest factor in weight loss or weight gain, if you're concerned with your overall well-being, understanding the details of how these foods affect your body is very important.

# Advantages of the Macronutrient Diet

The biggest selling point of the macronutrient diet is that this style of flexible dieting allows you to enjoy the foods you love, guilt-free. Well, as long as you account for them and make sure you don't overeat. It's been clearly shown that total energy balance, or calories in versus calories out, is what determines weight loss. There are no evil foods or special rules about how many meals you need to eat. Food you eat after six p.m. isn't automatically going to make you fat, and plenty of people have lost significant weight using a diet composed of mostly fast foods or processed snacks. Just because this works does not mean it's ideal. Sure, you can lose fat, but if you want your body to run at 100 percent efficiency and be healthy on the inside as well, it's important to make sure you're getting the right foods in your diet. Flexible dieting doesn't mean that you have to eat the fun foods and snacks; it just means that you can.

# Just What Is a Macronutrient Diet?

The macro diet, or flexible diet, simply refers to tracking your food, being precise with your macronutrient intake, and giving yourself the freedom to choose what foods you want to eat. Flexible dieting could be applied to carb cycling, a clean eating diet, the Paleo diet, a ketogenic diet, or any other diet, really.

# Eating for Maximum Health

You must understand that the "clean eating" diet isn't the only way to diet for maximum health. It's very possible, and in fact more sustainable in the long term, to eat the foods you enjoy in moderation on a regular basis. The idea of giving up any one food forever is a scary idea, but if you know you can enjoy your favorite foods whenever you want, guilt-free, so long as you account for them, it makes the prospect of long-term dieting much easier.

# Synergistic Nutrition

The most important reason for choosing whole foods is the micronutrients they contain. Micronutrients are the vitamins and minerals that support all of your body's important functions, like muscular contractions, mental functioning, and a healthy immune system. Without proper micronutrients, you may look fine on the outside, but you're not giving your body everything it needs to be healthy on the inside.

Vitamins and minerals can be obtained through pills and powders, but nothing works as well as getting them from your food. Many minerals work together to enhance each other, and whole foods often contain the vitamins and minerals that work well together.

# Psychological Benefits of the Macronutrient Diet

The number one benefit of this diet, and the reason so many people find it sustainable for the long haul, is the lack of restriction. It's not a free-for-all diet, and you do need to exercise some self-control and portion control, but you can still eat any food you want, so long as it fits your macro targets for the day.

# The Freedom to Choose

Freedom to choose what foods you want to eat is a refreshing approach to dieting, and the one that will be the most sustainable. Basic psychology reveals that humans tend to be more drawn to what they aren't supposed to have. If someone walked up and told you that you could never eat your favorite food again, how much more would you crave it? Even if you didn't want it that badly before, knowing it would be off the table forever would probably make you want it.

# Physical Benefits

From a physical health perspective, flexible dieting is a great way to get in shape and ensure you're getting the proper nutrients you need without any guesswork. The precision required means that if you set up your numbers and food sources properly, you can give your body exactly what it needs to feel and look good day after day. Other diets tend to take a broad approach; they ask you to eliminate certain food groups, try to control your portions, and hope for the best. Sometimes this works and sometimes it doesn't, but these other diets don't always ensure you're actually getting the right nutrients.

# Automate What Tracking You Can

To avoid getting stuck tracking your macros forever, it's best to automate as much as you can. Find one or two breakfasts you enjoy, one or two lunches you enjoy, and a few snacks. By cycling through these same meals over and over, you'll really only have to worry about measuring and tracking dinner, or whatever your free meal may be.

# Lifestyle Benefits

The number one benefit of the flexible diet is that as long as you track your macros, you can eat any foods you want at any time of the day, and if the numbers add up, you'll still see the changes in your body that you desire. No other diet out there allows this sort of customization to your individual lifestyle.

# Fill Up on Whole Foods

While you may understand that calories are what matter, you may not understand all the reasons why whole-food sources are more beneficial than packaged, processed foods. Before looking at the details of each macronutrient, you need to know why whole foods are important to include in your diet when it comes to helping you stay on track and make the right choices.

# When to Use Supplements

You don't need any supplements at all to lose weight. Certain supplements, like protein, fish oil, and vitamin D, can be very useful for overall health, but you can get enough from your diet if it's properly structured. If you're curious about a supplement, use Examine.com to find unbiased research reviews from doctors who will tell you if a given ingredient works, and if so, how much to use.

For an up-to-date list of supplements the author uses and recommends in his fitness coaching business, as well as bonus resources for readers, visit MattDustin.com/macronutrients.

# Be Nutritionally Accurate

Nutritional accuracy is very important when tracking macronutrients. If you plan to eat a variety of foods, throw in some treats from time to time, and still come close to your macro goals every day, you'd better know exactly what you're eating. Nutritional labels are usually close but are not 100 percent accurate, and there's no way to really know what you're getting. It's fine to eat foods out of packages, but then you're also getting a whole lot of other added, unnecessary ingredients.

# Prepare Your Own Meals

Whenever possible, prepare your own meals using whole-food ingredients. Even if your measurements aren't perfect, you'll still be in a much better place than simply hoping the restaurant calculations are accurate or existing solely off packaged snack foods.

# Macronutrients and Energy

There are three categories of energy systems in your body—complex processes that produce the required energy for whatever activity you're doing. Within these categories are various subcategories, but unless you're concerned with elite levels of human performance optimization, the subcategories aren't particularly important to understand. For fat loss and nutrition, you just need to know the basics of the big three systems. You'll learn what these three systems are and why they are important in the sections that follow.

# The Importance of Exercise

It's very important to look at exercise as a means of improving your body's health—because it is. If you see it as punishment or strictly as a way to burn calories, it will be much harder to enjoy it and make it a sustainable habit. Remember, you are getting stronger and setting yourself up to live a longer, healthier life. Burning extra calories is just a nice side effect.

# The Three Energy Systems in Your Body

Whether you're sleeping in bed or sprinting up a hill, one of the three energy systems is at work. The scientific names for these systems are the ATP-PC system, glycolytic system, and oxidative system, but just think of them as the fast, medium, and slow energy systems. For fat loss and nutrition, you just need to know the basics of the systems.

# The Fast Energy System

This fast energy system is your maximum effort, short-duration system. It can supply an intense burst of energy for around 10–12 seconds before it runs out of steam and the next system takes over. This is used when you are jumping, lifting something very heavy, or doing a fast and short run, like sprinting across a basketball court.

In terms of nutrition, you don't really need to worry about this one too much. Just know it exists. Because it's such a short burst of energy, it uses something called adenosine triphosphate (ATP), which is made and stored in your muscle cells. As long as you're getting enough calories and nutrients, you'll have plenty of ATP available.

# The Medium Energy System

Next up is the glycolytic system, or medium energy system, which is pretty complicated. All you need to know is that this system powers your moderate-to-high intensity, short-duration activities, such as sprinting, lifting weights, playing a sport, or anything else that would feel like a workout. The medium energy system kicks in after about 10 seconds, when the fast energy system runs out, and works for slightly longer—although it still runs out fairly quickly.

# Lifting Weights and Strength Training

When you lift weights or strength train, you create an environment where your body will be more inclined to use nutrients for recovery and repair rather than stored fat reserves. Resistance training causes micro damage to your muscles, and your body will be working hard for hours, even days, to repair the damage—a job that burns calories and requires carbs.

# Gluconeogenesis—Another Way to Get Glucose

So what happens if there is no glycogen in the muscles to be used? If you remember, you learned that carbohydrates are not essential for life. If they aren't essential, and you aren't consuming any and storing them as glycogen, how does this medium energy system operate? Well, your body can undergo the complex process of gluconeogenesis. This process involves breaking down stored muscle tissue, ripping it apart, and converting it to glucose. This is a much slower way to get glucose and is not optimal.

# Moving Into Recovery Mode

In addition to serving as fuel, carbohydrates play an important role in recovery from training and exercise. After a tough workout, your body switches into recovery mode, as it needs to work hard to repair the damage you did. This repair process requires energy, and giving your body carbs will allow it to do a better job of rebuilding the muscle tissue you broke down.

If you regularly exercise intensely, your best bet is including carbs in your diet, at least on workout days. You can work out without carbs, but your performance will suffer, as you won't have that glycogen ready for easy access. Think of your glycogen stores as a fuel tank for the car that is your body and carbohydrates as the fuel. Without fueling up, you'll have a difficult time operating at peak efficiency for any length of time.

# The Slow Energy System

The last of the big three you need to know about is the oxidative system. This is the slow energy system and provides a sustained release of energy for low-to-moderate activities that last a bit longer. Long runs, swimming, hiking, hot yoga, yard work—these are all activities that are more intense than your resting state but can be sustained for a long time. This system uses a mixture of carbohydrates and fats for fuel. While carbohydrates are still important and will benefit your body when it's using the oxidative system, they aren't quite as important as they are to the medium energy system.

# NEAT (Non-Exercise Activity Thermogenesis)

NEAT, or non-exercise activity thermogenesis, simply refers to the calories burned from any activity that wouldn't be considered traditional exercise. If you hate exercise, there are plenty of ways you can still increase your daily energy output. Park far away from your destination when you go places and walk more, try to stand up periodically throughout the day, and just move more as often as possible.

# Lean Body Mass

Your lean body mass is your total body weight minus body fat. It's very hard to calculate this number perfectly without advanced testing, but you can try. Figure out your body fat percentage from measuring using a handheld device, a digital scale that tracks body fat, or get a local trainer at your gym to measure your body fat. If none of these are options, you can search online for body fat measurement pictures. Your total body weight times your body fat percentage will tell you how many pounds of fat you carry, and your total weight minus fat calculation gives you your lean body mass weight.

# Meal Frequency Is Irrelevant

Meal frequency is mostly irrelevant for weight loss. You've probably read over and over that you need to eat four to five small meals spread evenly throughout the day. This simply isn't true. Studies have looked at multiple small meals compared to one or two large meals, and as long as the calories were the same, the results were the same.

# Flexible Dieting

With flexible dieting, you can build a meal plan that fits your schedule. If you find you have a very busy morning with no time to eat, you can grab a light snack and save most of your calories for later in the day. If you wake up starving, you can eat a huge breakfast. If you work split shifts or are a student with an irregular schedule, you can simply eat whenever you have a minute to sit down and make the numbers work. There is no rigid schedule or strict meal plan to follow. Every part of the macronutrient diet can be tailored to your exact needs and preferences.

# Fun Without Self-Sabotage

Carrying excess body fat is far more unhealthy than whatever trace ingredients might be in your afternoon snack. If someone is maintaining a healthy body weight with the occasional vending machine snack or diet soda thrown in, that person is much healthier than the person who's still forty pounds overweight and worrying about GMOs and artificial sweeteners. This book is meant to help you finally make a lasting change and not get caught up in the minor details. Worry about those little things later.

The truth is, the most effective diet is the one you can stick to for a long time. Making a lasting change takes time, and bouncing from diet to diet, losing and gaining the same five pounds over and over, isn't going to get you anywhere. If having a cookie every night after dinner helps you finally reach your goal weight, that's significantly better than trying to cut out all sweets and resorting to binge eating every weekend, making no long-term progress.

**5**

# Ingredients for a Healthy Macronutrient Diet

We've already looked at why macronutrients are essential to your body and how you can calculate how much protein, carbs, and fat you need in your diet to meet your goal. Now we're going to look at exactly how to build the best diet for you.

# Eating Junk Food

The macronutrient diet does not require you to eat junk food on a regular basis; it simply allows it. The macro diet, or flexible diet, simply refers to tracking your food, being precise with your macronutrient intake, and giving yourself the freedom to choose what foods you want to eat.

# Whole Food Instead of Processed Food

While there are many different supplements on the market that offer vitamin and mineral support, nothing beats the nutritional value of whole foods. Supplements can be a good safety net, but if that's your only source of these micros, you're not going to see the full benefit of consuming them. Whole foods contain natural combinations of these vitamins and minerals so they can work together in your body to be even more effective, which is a benefit individual supplements are unable to replicate.

# Variety Is the Spice of Life

Just because you eat a lot of vegetables doesn't mean you're getting enough micronutrients. It's the quality that matters, not the quantity. Eating chicken and broccoli three times a day may keep you well within your macronutrient targets, but you're getting only the nutrients from broccoli in that example. Don't fall into the bad habit of eating only a few vegetables; make an effort to eat as many as possible.

To help you get your nutrients in, here are a few strategies that can help you stay on track with your goals and ensure you're getting the right variety. Your diet may never be perfect, but you can always work to make it as healthy as possible.

# Eat the Rainbow

This isn't referring to a popular candy; it refers to eating all the colored fruits and vegetables you can get your hands on. Fruits and vegetables often get their color from micronutrients. For example, foods high in beta-carotene often appear orange, like carrots and sweet potatoes. Eating a wide variety of colorful vegetables sounds complicated to do, but it's easier than it seems. Keeping mixed bell peppers on hand, either fresh or frozen for stir-fries, is an easy way to get your red, green, yellow, and orange vegetables in. Combine them with some mixed berries for antioxidants with a few meals and plenty of leafy greens, like spinach, kale, and green cruciferous vegetables such as broccoli, and you'll be well on your way to a nutritious diet.

# Fruits or Veggies in Every Meal

If you find it hard to get enough fruits and vegetables in your diet, make it a habit to eat a serving of fruits or vegetables with every main meal. Oftentimes people will eat a salad or vegetables with dinner but opt for quick and easy meals for breakfast and lunch. That is fine, but there's always a way to add more nutritional value to your meals.

With breakfast, the easiest way to do this is by keeping fruit on hand. Oranges, apples, bananas, kiwis, berries, and pears are all very healthy fruits that are absolutely packed with nutrients. These fruits are easy to eat and can also be carried around for a quick and healthy snack throughout the day.

# Salads Are Your Friends

For lunch and dinner, salads and vegetables are your friend. It's very easy to throw several handfuls of mixed greens and spinach into a bowl, top with some low-fat dressing, and enjoy. Not only will this provide a large dose of antioxidants and nutrients, but it will keep you feeling full between meals. If you really struggle with this, a multivitamin or greens powder may be helpful, but those should never be your main source of nutrition, just a backup insurance policy. Make an effort to get your micronutrients in every single day, and your body will thank you.

# Poultry

With poultry like chicken and turkey, the quality isn't quite as important as their fat content. Whenever possible, go for the cuts with the least amount of fat possible. Lean ground turkey, lean turkey breast, and boneless, skinless chicken breasts are all great options.

Both chicken and turkey can be prepared with virtually zero added fat, which can be a nice alternative to beef products, which have fat that is much harder to remove. While the skin can be quite fatty, it's okay to enjoy it as long as you account for the fat. It's also very easy to cook chicken with the skin to retain the meat's moisture and flavor, and then just remove it before eating.

# Pork

When it comes to pork, try to stick to lean pork chops or pork loin. Other sources of pork like bacon or sausages are fine to eat, but they'll generally have high fat to protein ratios, which can make it a bit harder to fit into your daily macros. Many people tend to vilify pork, but if you choose a lean cut and prepare it correctly, it's perfectly fine to enjoy.

# Beef

Whenever possible, choose grass-fed beef sources. This costs a bit more, but the nutritional benefit is much better, and the flavor tends to be a bit richer and more powerful. There are several reasons why grass-fed beef is beneficial, and if you can make room for it in your budget, it's significantly better than farm-raised beef. Cows raised on farms are generally kept in small pens and fed grain-heavy diets, which can lead to beef that is lacking in nutrients. Cows that are free to graze on grass and move around a bit more will have more nutrients from all the greens and tend to provide leaner and healthier cuts of beef, as the cows get more exercise and fresh air. Grass-fed beef is high in omega-3 fatty acids, which are anti-inflammatory, as well as CLA, or conjugated linoleic acid, a fatty acid associated with healthy body fat levels.

# Fiber-Rich Carbs

When it comes to carbohydrates, the biggest concern is fiber content. High-fiber carbs, like oats, whole grains, and green vegetables, are excellent for your digestive system and keeping you full. Adequate fiber intake is also associated with improved heart health and blood sugar levels.

# Lean Proteins

Of all the nutrients, protein may be the most misunderstood. People are quick to vilify carbohydrates and fats, claiming they are all sorts of evil, but no one seems to know what to think about protein. Some say it damages your liver; others say you need incredibly high amounts of protein in your diet. The answer is somewhere in the middle. Protein in proper quantities won't have any negative effects, but you probably don't need as much as most people claim. For optimal recovery from training, satiety, and a healthy body, 1 gram of protein per pound of lean body weight is a pretty good guideline.

# The Macronutrient Diet Works with Any Goal

A flexible diet is adaptable to any lifestyle and schedule. Where most diets are focused solely on fat loss, the macronutrient diet works with any goal, whether that goal is fat loss, muscle gain, athletic performance, or simply general health. The next section will provide real-life examples of how this diet can be the perfect fit for any lifestyle. It may sound too good to be true; after all, diets aren't supposed to be fun, right? Well, not only can this diet be fun, but it's also the best option for a sustainable, healthy plan that you could realistically follow for the rest of your life. Most diets are too restrictive and aren't meant to last longer than twelve weeks. If you put in the time to understand and learn how flexible dieting works, you'll know how to eat for optimal health for the rest of your life.

# Keep It In Balance

By now you should understand that fat is not evil; rather, it's a necessary component of a diet for optimal long-term health. The right sources of fat keep your hormones functioning, your brain operating on all cylinders, your skin healthy, and your joints and cells protected. Fat is important. Not all fat is good, however. While you should be adding fat to your diet, it's vital to make sure you're getting the right fats in the right balances. Refer to Chapter 2 for a closer look at the various types of fat, where they come from, and how to properly balance them. As a refresher, it's important to understand the benefits of healthy fats, just to make sure you aren't still scared of enjoying them.

# Make a Diet and Stick with It

The truth is, the most effective diet is the one you can stick to for a long time. Making a lasting change takes time, and bouncing from diet to diet, losing and gaining the same five pounds over and over, isn't going to get you anywhere. If having a cookie every night after dinner helps you finally reach your goal weight, that's significantly better than trying to cut out all sweets and resorting to binge eating every weekend, making no long-term progress.

# Problems with Processed Food

The issue with eating processed foods is that they are generally lacking in micronutrients. Spending your macros on processed foods means you'll have less available for whole foods that provide those good nutrients. Many people try to use a multivitamin or greens supplement as nutritional insurance, which isn't a bad idea, but nothing will be as good as eating whole foods every day.

# The 80/20 Rule

Most people find they are able to manage their nutrition while still enjoying themselves by following the 80/20 rule of nutrition. This means that 80 percent of the time you choose healthy food sources to the best of your ability. The other 20 percent of the time you enjoy what would traditionally be considered "bad" foods—your favorite dessert, a few drinks, or a slice of pizza, for example.

# 6

# 50+ Macronutrient Recipes

Here are more than fifty macronutrient-rich recipes that are flavorful, easy to make, and delicious! They're a mixture of traditional and vegetarian, including such favorites as Shrimp Ceviche Salad, Chicken and Pesto Farfalle, and Garlic Cheddar Cauliflower Soup. From breakfasts to dinner with soups, salads, and snacks in between, every meal is covered. And of course, there's always room for desserts like Triple-Berry Yogurt Parfait and Frozen Chocolate Bananas.

# Low-Carb Protein Waffle

*This tasty breakfast will satisfy your cravings without giving you any unneces-*
*sary carbohydrates. Choose a protein flavor you like, as this will influence the*
*final flavor.*

## Serves 1

1 (30-gram) scoop whey protein (any
flavor)
1 teaspoon baking powder

1 teaspoon cinnamon
1 large egg
½ cup water

1.  Preheat a waffle maker for 5 minutes.
2.  Add whey protein, baking powder, and cinnamon to a medium bowl and mix well.
3.  Add egg and mix well with a fork.
4.  Add water and mix well; more can be added to reach your desired consistency.
5.  Cook 45–60 seconds in the waffle maker and serve immediately.

**PER SERVING**

Calories: 185 | Fat: 5g | Protein: 31g | Sodium: 602mg | Fiber: 1.5g |
Carbohydrates: 5g | Sugar: 1g

### Top It with Flavor

This waffle is very low calorie and can be topped with butter, whipped cream, syrup,
fresh fruit, or any other topping you love. If you have higher carbs on waffle day, top it
with fresh fruit and maybe some natural maple syrup. If it's a low-carb day, you can top
it with some nut butters or whipped cream to add some flavor and nutrition.

# Peaches and Cream Oatmeal

*This spin on a classic dish is a refreshing breakfast for those hot summer mornings, and it packs a protein punch.*

## Serves 1

1¼ cups water
½ cup dry quick-cooking oats
1 (30-gram) scoop vanilla whey
   protein

½ cup skim milk
1 (1-gram) packet stevia
1 medium peach, peeled, pitted, and
   sliced

1. Combine water and oats in a medium microwave-safe bowl.
2. Cook in microwave on high 3 minutes or until desired texture is reached.
3. In a separate bowl or shaker cup, mix protein and milk, then add to the cooked oats and stir. Add stevia and mix well.
4. Top with peaches and serve immediately.

### PER SERVING

Calories: 368 | Fat: 4.5g | Protein: 36g | Sodium: 105mg | Fiber: 6g |
Carbohydrates: 51g | Sugar: 20g

### The Power of Oatmeal

Oatmeal is very high in fiber, so it will keep you feeling full all morning long while providing a slow, sustained release of energy. Because of its fiber content, oatmeal can absorb a lot of water, so be sure to stay hydrated and drink one to two big glasses of water with each serving.

# Chocolate Protein French Toast

*French toast is traditionally loaded with calories. This version provides the protein, carbs, and fats you need for a balanced meal.*

## Serves 1

Nonstick cooking spray
3 large egg whites
½ (30-gram) scoop chocolate protein powder

2 slices whole-grain bread
1 (1-gram) packet stevia
1 teaspoon cinnamon
½ cup sugar-free maple syrup

1. Heat a medium skillet over medium-high heat and coat lightly with cooking spray.
2. Whisk together egg whites and protein in a large bowl.
3. Dip bread into egg and protein mixture, coating both sides.
4. Add slices to skillet, cooking 2–3 minutes per side or until golden brown.
5. Remove from skillet; top with stevia, cinnamon, and syrup. Serve immediately.

**PER SERVING**
Calories: 295 | Fat: 2g | Protein: 29g | Sodium: 689mg | Fiber: 3g | Carbohydrates: 46g | Sugar: 7g

### The Best Bread?

When choosing a bread, look for a whole-grain, multigrain, or sprouted bread. The calories will be similar to white bread, but you'll be getting more fiber and other beneficial nutrients. The high fiber content can also help with feelings of fullness and satiety between meals.

# Low-Carb Southwestern Egg Wrap

*By skipping the tortilla, you can use eggs to add healthy fats and proteins to your meal while lowering your carb intake.*

**Serves 1**

1½ teaspoons butter
2 large eggs
1 tablespoon skim milk
2 slices bacon, cooked and crumbled
½ medium avocado, peeled, pitted, and sliced

¼ cup shredded Mexican cheese
½ teaspoon salt
½ teaspoon freshly ground black pepper
½ cup fresh salsa

1. Heat a medium skillet over medium-high heat and coat lightly with butter.
2. Mix eggs and milk in a small bowl with a fork and pour into heated pan.
3. Cook 1–2 minutes per side, flipping when edges start to peel off the pan.
4. Plate eggs, and add bacon, avocado, and cheese before rolling into a burrito shape.
5. Season with salt and pepper, top with salsa, and serve.

**PER SERVING**
Calories: 731 | Fat: 60g | Protein: 32g | Sodium: 2,916mg | Fiber: 8g | Carbohydrates: 19g | Sugar: 8g

## Make Your Own Salsa

Salsa is an incredibly versatile and low-calorie snack that goes well with anything. You can top meat, eggs, or any Mexican dish with salsa, or enjoy it plain. Store-bought salsas are fine, but it's very easy to make at home, and there are countless recipes. The easiest base recipe is 2 chopped medium tomatoes, ½ chopped medium onion, 2 tablespoons cilantro, chopped, and 1 tablespoon minced garlic. From there, add any flavor enhancers or extra ingredients that you enjoy.

# Avocado Toast

*This combo is perfect for meeting your daily carb quota, and the fat content will help slow down digestion so you don't experience an energy spike and abrupt crash from the toast. For an extra protein boost, you can top this recipe with fried or scrambled eggs.*

## Serves 1

1 medium avocado, peeled, pitted, and mashed

1 teaspoon garlic salt

1 teaspoon freshly ground black pepper

2 slices whole-grain bread

1. In a medium bowl, combine avocado, garlic salt, and pepper.
2. Toast bread to desired doneness and spread avocado mixture on each slice before serving.

**PER SERVING**

Calories: 398 | Fat: 24g | Protein: 8g | Sodium: 2,621mg | Fiber: 12g | Carbohydrates: 43g | Sugar: 4g

# Superfood Breakfast Bowl

*This high-carb recipe is loaded with micronutrients. This is the perfect fuel-up meal for high-activity days, as the carbohydrates and fiber will keep you full while providing electrolytes to keep you hydrated and energized during physical activity.*

## Serves 2

½ cup unsweetened plain almond milk

½ teaspoon cinnamon

½ teaspoon vanilla extract

¼ cup uncooked quinoa

1 medium banana, sliced

6 strawberries, sliced

½ cup blueberries

2 teaspoons hemp seeds

1. In a small saucepan, bring almond milk, cinnamon, and vanilla to a boil.
2. Stir in quinoa, reduce to a simmer, and cook 20 minutes or until desired consistency is reached.
3. Top with banana, berries, and hemp seeds. Enjoy warm.

**PER SERVING**

Calories: 200 | Fat: 4g | Protein: 6g | Sodium: 43mg | Fiber: 6g | Carbohydrates: 38g | Sugar: 14g

# Cilantro Chicken and Avocado Burritos

*If you have precooked chicken available, this recipe can be assembled in minutes. Use grilled or roasted chicken strips from the store, or make your own using your favorite chicken recipe.*

## Serves 4

1 pound skinless chicken, cooked and shredded

1 medium avocado, peeled, pitted, and diced

1 cup shredded Mexican cheese

1 cup salsa verde

½ cup sour cream

4 tablespoons chopped cilantro

4 large tortillas

1. Equally distribute all ingredients between tortillas.
2. Roll up tortillas to form burritos and serve.

**PER SERVING**

Calories: 497 | Fat: 26g | Protein: 35g | Sodium: 632mg | Fiber: 4g | Carbohydrates: 31g | Sugar: 4g

### Rotate Your Chicken

These burritos can be assembled with any sort of precooked chicken (served warm or cold). Many grocery stores sell precooked chicken, either whole or already sliced. If you're running short on time, this is an excellent shortcut. You can use it plain or add any seasoning or sauce you want to keep the flavor interesting.

# California Roll in a Bowl

*The California roll may be the most popular sushi roll in America, and the ingredients are quite simple. If you want a sushi fix but don't want to learn how to roll it yourself, this bowl is a quick and easy way to enjoy some fresh California roll.*

## Serves 2

2 cups cooked white rice
½ cup chopped imitation crab
½ medium cucumber, peeled and chopped
½ medium avocado, peeled, pitted, and sliced

1 sheet dried seaweed, crumbled
1 tablespoon toasted sesame seeds
¼ cup soy sauce
¼ cup rice vinegar
¼ cup pickled sushi ginger

1. Combine all ingredients except soy sauce, vinegar, and ginger in a large bowl and mix well.
2. Evenly divide mixture into two serving bowls.
3. In a separate container, mix soy sauce and vinegar.
4. Drizzle sauce over rice mixture, top with ginger, and serve.

### PER SERVING

Calories: 437 | Fat: 8g | Protein: 13g | Sodium: 2,450mg | Fiber: 4g | Carbohydrates: 78g | Sugar: 14g

# Shrimp Ceviche Salad

*This is a quick and easy dish that packs lean protein and healthy fats. You can enjoy this salad as is or, if you want some extra carbs, try serving it with tortilla chips for dipping.*

## Serves 2

1 large avocado, peeled, pitted, and diced
2 green onion stalks, chopped
1 (4-ounce) can salad shrimp
1 medium tomato, diced
3 tablespoons chopped cilantro
1 teaspoon salt
1 teaspoon freshly ground black pepper
Juice from ½ medium lime

1. Add all ingredients except lime juice to a large bowl. Gently toss until mixed well, being careful not to smash the avocado chunks too much.
2. Divide into two medium bowls, top each with a drizzle of lime juice, and serve.

**PER SERVING**
Calories: 223 | Fat: 14g | Protein: 14g | Sodium: 1,663mg | Fiber: 8g | Carbohydrates: 16g | Sugar: 3g

### Canned Seafood
While canned seafoods like tuna, crab, or shrimp may not be quite as tasty and nutritious as their fresh alternatives, they are a quick and easy source of ready-to-go protein. Try not to get all of your seafood from a can, but when you want something convenient and quick, like in this recipe, canned seafood is an excellent option to have around.

# Tuna Salad

*This protein-packed recipe is perfect for when you need a quick meal. You can enjoy it as a traditional sandwich, a tortilla wrap, or plain if you're watching your carbs.*

## Serves 4

2 (6-ounce) cans tuna packed in water

¼ teaspoon freshly ground black pepper

1 tablespoon olive oil

½ small red onion, peeled and thinly sliced

¼ cup roughly chopped kalamata olives

1. Drain and rinse tuna, removing any excess water.
2. In a medium bowl, combine tuna, pepper, oil, onion, and olives. Mix well and enjoy.

**PER SERVING**

Calories: 208 | Fat: 10g | Protein: 25g | Sodium: 351mg | Fiber: 0g | Carbohydrates: 3g | Sugar: 0g

# Buffalo Chicken Mini Wraps

*These bite-sized wraps are the perfect lunch. Once prepared, you can grab one anytime you need it, and you can wrap the mix in lettuce leaves instead of tortillas if you don't want the carbs.*

## Makes 15 wraps

3 large boneless, skinless chicken breasts, cut into ½" cubes
¾ cup Frank's RedHot Original Cayenne Pepper Sauce, divided
Nonstick cooking spray

1 medium avocado, peeled, pitted, and diced
15 mini tortillas
½ cup low-fat ranch dressing

1. Place chicken in a large bowl or resealable bag. Pour ½ cup hot sauce over chicken and marinate 1–2 hours in the refrigerator.
2. When ready to cook, heat a large skillet over medium heat, lightly coat with cooking spray, and cook chicken 10–12 minutes or until fully cooked through.
3. Add remaining hot sauce to cooked chicken, toss, and let cool 5 minutes.
4. Equally divide chicken and avocado between tortillas, drizzle with dressing, and serve.

**PER SERVING (1 WRAP)**

Calories: 170 | Fat: 5g | Protein: 14g | Sodium: 728mg | Fiber: 1g | Carbohydrates: 16g | Sugar: 2g

# Turkey Reuben Sandwiches

*A Reuben is traditionally a high-calorie meal, but this version drastically lowers the high-fat content typically found in Reubens.*

## Serves 2

1 tablespoon olive oil
4 ounces sliced turkey
2 slices reduced-fat Swiss cheese
½ cup sauerkraut, drained

¼ cup fat-free Thousand Island dressing
4 slices rye bread

1. Heat oil in a nonstick skillet over medium heat.
2. While pan heats, evenly divide turkey, cheese, sauerkraut, and dressing between the slices of rye bread, stacking two with toppings, then topping with the remaining two slices.
3. Cook sandwich in skillet 3–4 minutes per side, until bread is toasted and warm, then serve.

**PER SERVING**
Calories: 403 | Fat: 15g | Protein: 23g | Sodium: 1,502mg | Fiber: 6g | Carbohydrates:  43g | Sugar: 9g

## Sauerkraut and Your Gut
Fermented foods like sauerkraut provide an excellent source of live probiotics, which are essential for a healthy gut. Having the proper balance of good bacteria, which are found in fermented foods like sauerkraut, kimchi, and certain kinds of yogurt, will help maintain a healthy gut environment. A healthy gut strengthens your immune system and keeps your digestive system functioning.

# Turkey and Spinach Focaccia Sandwich

*This sandwich provides lean protein from the turkey, as well as micronutrients from the spinach and tomatoes. For added flavor and texture, lightly toast the focaccia bread slices before preparing.*

**Serves 2**

2 tablespoons low-fat mayonnaise
2 tablespoons chopped fresh basil
2 tablespoons sun-dried tomatoes
¼ teaspoon crushed red pepper

8 ounces sliced turkey
1 cup spinach leaves
4 slices focaccia bread

1. In a small bowl, mix mayonnaise, basil, tomatoes, and crushed red pepper. Divide the mixture in half.
2. Build sandwiches by layering the spread, turkey, and spinach leaves on two slices focaccia, and then topping with two slices.

**PER SERVING**
Calories: 421 | Fat: 13g | Protein: 25g | Sodium: 1,679mg | Fiber: 1g | Carbohydrates: 52g | Sugar: 3g

## Which Bread Should You Choose?

In terms of pure calories, there isn't a huge variety among bread manufacturers. You'll likely find most slices range from 80–140 calories. For maximum health, however, a sprouted whole-grain bread will be full of fiber and beneficial nutrients.

# Egg Salad

*Egg salad is a very versatile dish that can be served on a sandwich, added to a salad, or enjoyed as a side dish that's loaded with fat and protein.*

## Serves 4

8 large eggs
½ cup low-fat mayonnaise
1 teaspoon mustard
¼ cup chopped green onion
¼ teaspoon salt
¼ teaspoon freshly ground black pepper
¼ teaspoon paprika

1. Place eggs in a medium saucepan and add cold water until eggs are covered by 1" water.
2. Bring water to a boil, then immediately remove pan from heat. Cover and let eggs cook 10–12 minutes, then immediately drain and cool under running cold water.
3. Peel eggs, chop, and mix with mayonnaise, mustard, onion, and seasonings.

**PER SERVING**
Calories: 176 | Fat: 12g | Protein: 13g | Sodium: 559mg | Fiber: 0g | Carbohydrates: 5g | Sugar: 3g

# Pesto Chili

*This recipe contains a variety of beans to help make sure you get as many different essential amino acids and proteins in your diet as possible.*

## Serves 4

1 tablespoon olive oil
2 medium carrots, peeled and diced
1 small yellow onion, peeled and chopped
1 (15-ounce) can diced tomatoes
1 teaspoon salt
1 teaspoon freshly ground black pepper

2 cups water
1 (15-ounce) can chickpeas, drained and rinsed
1 (15-ounce) can cannellini beans, drained and rinsed
1 (15-ounce) can kidney beans, drained and rinsed
½ cup pesto

1. Add 1 tablespoon oil, carrots, and onion to a large saucepan over high heat and cook 3–5 minutes or until carrots are tender.
2. Stir in tomatoes, salt, pepper, and water and bring to a boil. Add chickpeas and other cans of beans, cooking until heated through (about 3 minutes).
3. Divide into 4 equal portions, top with pesto, and serve.

**PER SERVING**
Calories: 537 | Fat: 39g | Protein: 11g | Sodium: 1,209mg | Fiber: 12g | Carbohydrates: 37g | Sugar: 6g

### Mix Your Beans for Proper Protein
One of the biggest challenges with following a vegan or vegetarian diet can be getting adequate protein. Even if your goal isn't to build muscle, you need protein to live and function. While beans contain some protein, they don't necessarily have all the essential amino acids you need to get in your diet. Combining bean sources is a good way to make sure you're getting a variety of amino acids.

# Linguine and Caper Sauce

*This traditional Mediterranean-style pasta is simple to prepare and can be made in bulk in order to have reheated meals throughout the week.*

## Serves 6

1 tablespoon olive oil
2 cloves garlic, minced
¼ teaspoon red pepper flakes
1 (26-ounce) jar marinara sauce

1 (3.5-ounce) jar capers, chopped
½ cup chopped fresh parsley
½ teaspoon lemon zest
1 (16-ounce) package linguine

1. Combine oil, garlic, and red pepper flakes in a large saucepan over medium heat and cook 2 minutes until garlic becomes fragrant.
2. Stir in marinara, capers, parsley, and lemon zest, then reduce heat to low and simmer 15 minutes.
3. While sauce is simmering, prepare linguine according to the package directions.
4. Combine pasta and sauce, tossing until mixed well, and serve.

**PER SERVING**
Calories: 364 | Fat: 5g | Protein: 12g | Sodium: 900mg | Fiber: 5g | Carbohydrates: 66g | Sugar: 9g

# Avocado Southwestern Salad

*This filling, Southwestern-style salad is packed with healthy fats from the avocado and beans and makes the perfect side dish or stand-alone meal.*

## Serves 4

¼ cup olive oil
¼ cup lime juice
½ teaspoon ground cumin
1 teaspoon salt
1 teaspoon freshly ground black pepper
2 bags (about 12 cups) romaine lettuce

2 medium avocados, peeled, pitted, and cubed
1 (15.5-ounce) can pinto beans, drained and rinsed
1 cup cooked corn kernels
½ medium red onion, peeled and diced
½ cup chopped fresh cilantro

1. For dressing: Whisk together oil, lime juice, cumin, salt, and pepper until emulsified.
2. For salad: Toss lettuce, avocados, beans, corn, onion, and cilantro in a large bowl.
3. Mix dressing with salad and serve.

**PER SERVING**

Calories: 274 | Fat: 15g | Protein: 8g | Sodium: 882mg | Fiber: 9g | Carbohydrates: 32g | Sugar: 5g

# Pasta with Pesto and Olive Sauce

*This light and healthy dish uses fresh herbs and spices to make a very simple, low-fat recipe. If you want to get your carbs in without feeling weighed down, this is the light meal recipe for you.*

## Serves 4

1 (16-ounce) package spaghetti
½ cup reserved pasta water
2 cloves garlic
¼ cup olive oil
¼ cup green olives

¼ cup fresh parsley
¼ cup fresh basil
¼ cup black olives
½ teaspoon salt

1. Cook spaghetti al dente according to package directions and drain, reserving ½ cup pasta water.
2. For pesto: Combine garlic, oil, green olives, parsley, and basil in a blender and blend thoroughly.
3. Transfer pesto to a large saucepan and heat 2 minutes over medium heat until warm.
4. Add spaghetti, black olives, salt, and reserved water to the saucepan and continue cooking until water is absorbed and spaghetti is heated. Serve immediately.

**PER SERVING**

Calories: 320 | Fat: 17g | Protein: 7g | Sodium: 418mg | Fiber: 3g | Carbohydrates: 36g | Sugar: 1g

## Bump Up the Protein with Meat Substitutes

If you're looking to add more protein to meatless dishes, such as this pasta dish, consider adding tofu or tempeh. They are alternatives to protein derived from the soybean, and are an easy way to add some extra protein to your meals, replacing traditional proteins like seafood or meat.

# Black Bean Soup

*This soup requires a slow cooker, but leftovers can be stored in the refrigerator and reheated whenever you need an easy, protein-packed lunch.*

## Serves 6

2 tablespoons olive oil
2 medium carrots, peeled and chopped
2 stalks celery, chopped
1 medium onion, peeled and chopped
¼ cup tomato paste

3 cloves garlic, minced
1½ teaspoons ground cumin
3 (15-ounce) cans black beans, drained and rinsed
1 cup frozen or canned corn
3 cups vegetable broth

1. Heat oil in a medium skillet over medium-high heat.
2. Add carrots, celery, and onion to the pan and cook 5 minutes, stirring occasionally.
3. Stir in tomato paste, garlic, and cumin and continue to cook 2 minutes, stirring frequently.
4. In a large slow cooker (at least 4 quarts), combine skillet mixture with beans, corn, and broth. Cook on high 4 hours.
5. Serve warm or allow to cool and refrigerate for later.

**PER SERVING**
Calories: 293 | Fat: 7g | Protein: 14g | Sodium: 1,512mg | Fiber: 12g | Carbohydrates: 44g | Sugar: 11g

---

### Quinoa, the Complete Protein
On a vegetarian diet, it's very important to ensure you are getting complete protein sources that have all the amino acids you need. Quinoa is one of the most complete protein sources in the plant world and should be a staple in your diet.

# Meatless Cheddar Squash Casserole

*This casserole provides important nutrients and fiber from the squash, as well as protein from the milk, cheese, and eggs.*

## Serves 10

4 cups sliced summer squash
½ cup chopped onion
½ cup water
35 buttery round crackers, crushed
1 cup shredded Cheddar cheese
2 large eggs

¾ cup skim milk
1 teaspoon salt
½ teaspoon freshly ground black pepper
¼ cup unsalted butter, melted

1. Preheat oven to 400°F.
2. Place squash, onion, and water in a large skillet over medium-high heat and cover. Cook 5 minutes or until squash is tender, then drain and set aside.
3. In a medium bowl, combine crackers and cheese until well blended.
4. Stir half the cracker mixture into cooked squash and onions, mixing well.
5. In a separate medium bowl, whisk eggs and milk until well blended. Add to cracker and squash mixture, along with salt, pepper, and melted butter, mixing well.
6. Spread into a greased 9" × 13" glass baking dish, and top with remaining half of cracker and cheese mix.
7. Bake 25 minutes or until lightly browned, then serve.

**PER SERVING**
Calories: 184 | Fat: 13g | Protein: 7g | Sodium: 423mg | Fiber: 1g | Carbohydrates: 10g | Sugar: 3g

# Chickpea Salad

*This quick and easy chickpea salad can be enjoyed on a sandwich, in a wrap, or on top of a salad.*

## Serves 4

1 (19-ounce) can chickpeas, drained and rinsed
1 stalk celery, chopped
½ medium onion, peeled and chopped
1 tablespoon mayonnaise
1 tablespoon lemon juice
1 teaspoon dried dill

1. In a medium bowl mash chickpeas with a fork.
2. Add all other ingredients, mix well, and refrigerate until ready to eat.

**PER SERVING**
Calories: 125 | Fat: 4.2g | Protein: 5.2g | Sodium: 33mg | Fiber: 4.7g | Carbohydrates: 17.4g | Sugar: 3.5g

# Zucchini and Potato Bake

*Potatoes are full of important nutrients and are a very filling source of carbohydrates. Combined with zucchini, this nutritious and tasty recipe will keep you full for hours.*

## Serves 4

2 medium zucchini, sliced
4 medium potatoes, peeled and cut into large chunks
1 medium red bell pepper, seeded and chopped
1 clove garlic, minced

½ cup bread crumbs
¼ cup olive oil
1 teaspoon paprika
1 teaspoon salt
1 teaspoon freshly ground black pepper

1. Preheat oven to 400°F.
2. In a medium baking pan, toss all ingredients together, spreading evenly over the pan.
3. Bake 1 hour or until potatoes are tender, stirring occasionally.

**PER SERVING**

Calories: 349.65 | Fat: 14.9g | Protein: 7g | Sodium: 710mg | Fiber: 7.6g | Carbohydrates: 48g | Sugar: 7g

# Seared Chilean Sea Bass with Homemade Pesto

*This light and tasty recipe uses Chilean sea bass to pack in healthy proteins and fats, but the homemade pesto can be used on any whitefish for a delicious dinner.*

**Serves 4**

2 cups baby spinach
½ cup fresh parsley
1 clove garlic, smashed
¼ cup chopped walnuts
2 teaspoons fresh lemon juice
¼ cup plus 1 tablespoon extra-virgin olive oil, divided

1 teaspoon salt, divided
½ teaspoon freshly ground black pepper, divided
4 (6-ounce) pieces wild-caught Chilean sea bass

1. For pesto: Combine spinach, parsley, garlic, walnuts, lemon juice, ¼ cup oil, ½ teaspoon salt, and ¼ teaspoon pepper in a food processor and blend until smooth.
2. For sea bass: Heat remaining 1 tablespoon oil in a cast iron skillet over medium-high heat.
3. When oil just begins to smoke, season sea bass lightly with remaining salt and pepper and sear 3 minutes per side.
4. Remove from skillet, top with pesto, and serve.

**PER SERVING**
Calories: 358 | Fat: 32g | Protein: 14.8g | Sodium: 73.127mg | Fiber: 1g | Carbohydrates: 2.434g | Sugar: 0.386g

# Garlic and Herb-Roasted Salmon with Tomatoes

*Of all the fish, salmon is one of the healthiest, providing good omega-3 fatty acids that act as an anti-inflammatory and improve mental functioning.*

**Serves 4**

2 tablespoons extra-virgin olive oil
2 cloves garlic, minced
⅛ teaspoon cayenne pepper
1 teaspoon lemon juice
¼ cup chopped fresh parsley

1 teaspoon salt
4 wild-caught salmon fillets (about
   2 pounds)
12 cherry tomatoes
1 medium lemon, sliced into rounds

1. Preheat oven to 450°F.
2. In a small mixing bowl, combine oil, garlic, cayenne, lemon juice, parsley, and salt, mixing well.
3. Lay salmon skin-down on a baking sheet lined with parchment paper. Arrange cherry tomatoes and lemon slices between fillets.
4. Drizzle the fillets, lemon slices, and tomatoes with herb mixture.
5. Cook 6–8 minutes or until salmon is mostly done. Finish under the broiler 5 additional minutes to roast the lemons and tomatoes.
6. Remove and serve salmon with roasted lemon and tomatoes.

**PER SERVING**
Calories: 388.48 | Fat: 21g | Protein: 44.98g | Sodium: 692mg | Fiber: 0.622g | Carbohydrates: 2.3g | Sugar: 1.06g

### Choose Your Fish Wisely
When choosing fish, opt for wild-caught whenever possible. Wild-caught fish are much higher in good fats, and you can even find wild-caught fish canned and ready to eat if you don't live near an ocean or lake where fresh fish is usually plentiful.

# Crispy Parmesan Tilapia

*While tilapia is low in fat, it is also a very cheap source of protein. Due to its mild flavor, it is easy to use in a variety of recipes. This crispy tilapia recipe can be served with your favorite salad or pasta.*

## Serves 4

1 cup Italian bread crumbs
¼ cup chopped fresh parsley
1 cup freshly grated Parmesan cheese
½ teaspoon salt

¼ cup lemon juice
4 (4-ounce) tilapia fillets
4 cloves garlic, minced
¼ teaspoon red pepper flakes
2 tablespoons olive oil

1. Preheat oven to 400°F.
2. Mix bread crumbs, parsley, Parmesan, and salt in a shallow bowl or serving dish.
3. Place lemon juice in a separate shallow dish and coat tilapia in it. Next, coat fish in the bread crumb mixture before transferring to a lightly oiled baking sheet.
4. Top fillets with garlic and red pepper flakes, and drizzle or spray with oil to help it crisp.
5. Bake 10–12 minutes until fully cooked, then serve.

**PER SERVING**
Calories: 185.69 | Fat: 10.2g | Protein: 24.98g | Sodium: 858.34mg | Fiber: 1.49g | Carbohydrates: 21.71g | Sugar: 2.11g

### The Leanest Fish?
In general, whitefish like cod, halibut, and tilapia are lower in fat and are a good choice when you're watching your calories. High-fat fish, like tuna or salmon, have more calories but also more good omega-3 fatty acids. The choice is yours.

# Clam Chowder

*This hearty, traditional New England–style clam chowder is very filling and provides a good mix of protein, carbs, and fat. You can double the recipe to make a large batch to store in bulk.*

## Serves 4

1 tablespoon canola oil
1 medium celery root, peeled and chopped
2 large carrots, peeled and chopped
2 stalks celery, chopped
2 large potatoes, peeled and chopped
1 large onion, peeled and chopped
¼ teaspoon salt

¼ teaspoon freshly ground black pepper
1 (8-ounce) bottle clam juice
2 cups water
2 tablespoons cornstarch
1 cup skim milk
2 (6-ounce) cans baby clams
1 cup cooked corn kernels

1. Add oil, celery root, carrots, celery, potatoes, onion, salt, and pepper to a large stockpot. Cover and cook 12 minutes over medium heat until onions and potatoes are softened.
2. Add clam juice and water. Return to a boil over high heat, then reduce to low heat and simmer 20–25 minutes.
3. In a separate small dish, mix cornstarch and milk until starch is fully dissolved. Add mixture to soup and stir until well blended.
4. Add clams and corn. Continue to cook 5 more minutes, then serve.

**PER SERVING**

Calories: 264.78 | Fat: 4.757g | Protein: 7.14g | Sodium: 364mg | Fiber: 7.2g | Carbohydrates: 50.93g | Sugar: 9.941g

# Lemon-Steamed Halibut

*This simple and citrusy dish works well with halibut but can also be prepared with cod, tilapia, or any other whitefish instead.*

### Serves 6

6 (4-ounce) halibut fillets
1 tablespoon dried dill
1 tablespoon onion powder
2 teaspoons dried parsley
¼ teaspoon paprika

¼ teaspoon salt
¼ teaspoon lemon pepper
¼ teaspoon garlic powder
2 tablespoons lemon juice

1. Preheat oven to 375°F.
2. Cut six foil squares big enough to fold each fillet into its own foil packet.
3. Place a fillet on each foil square and sprinkle with dill, onion powder, parsley, paprika, salt, lemon pepper, and garlic powder, then drizzle fillets with lemon juice.
4. Fold foil around each fillet to create a sealed packet. Place packets on a large baking sheet.
5. Bake 20–25 minutes until fish flakes easily with a fork.

**PER SERVING**
Calories: 130.58 | Fat: 2.635g | Protein: 23.622g | Sodium: 162mg | Fiber: 0.35g | Carbohydrates: 1.7g | Sugar: 0.221g

### Choose Your Fish

There's a wide variety of fish to choose from, all with their own unique flavors and nutritional profiles. If you're used to sticking with the basics, like tilapia and tuna, try some of the other options available at your local store. Red snapper, cod, Chilean sea bass, or any of the other fish you may find are excellent to try in this recipe.

# Shrimp Taco Salad

*If fish tacos aren't your thing, this spicy Southwestern-style Shrimp Taco Salad may be right up your alley. Packed with healthy fats, proteins, and micronutrients, this is the perfect summer dinner.*

## Serves 4

¼ cup lime juice
2 tablespoons olive oil
1 teaspoon ground cumin
2 teaspoons minced garlic
2 teaspoons chipotle hot sauce
¾ pound medium shrimp, peeled and deveined

1 cup chopped romaine lettuce
½ cup chopped green onions
¼ cup chopped fresh cilantro
1 (15-ounce) can black beans, drained and rinsed
3 plum tomatoes, chopped
2 cups crushed tortilla chips

1. Preheat grill to medium-high.
2. Combine lime juice, oil, cumin, garlic, and hot sauce in a small bowl and set aside.
3. Place shrimp on metal grill skewers and lightly drizzle with 1 tablespoon of lime juice mixture. Grill shrimp skewers 4 minutes per side.
4. Place grilled shrimp in a large bowl and add lettuce, onions, cilantro, black beans, and tomatoes, tossing well with remaining lime mixture.
5. Evenly divide tortilla chips between four bowls, top with shrimp salad, and serve.

**PER SERVING**

Calories: 247.43 | Fat: 9.09g | Protein: 22.95g | Sodium: 477.33mg | Fiber: 6.22g | Carbohydrates: 18.35g | Sugar: 3.7g

# Maryland Crab Cakes

*These traditional Baltimore favorites are a delicious and easy-to-prepare meal that can be enjoyed plain, served as a side dish, or made into a sandwich.*

## Makes 6 cakes

2 slices white bread, crusts trimmed
1 pound crabmeat (available in cans at most stores)
1 large egg
1 tablespoon mayonnaise

1 teaspoon Dijon mustard
1 teaspoon Worcestershire sauce
1 tablespoon Old Bay Seasoning or other seafood seasoning
2 tablespoons butter

1. Rip bread into small pieces and add to a large bowl with crab, egg, mayonnaise, mustard, Worcestershire sauce, and Old Bay, mixing gently with a large spoon or by hand.
2. Shape mixture into six round patties and set aside.
3. Heat butter in a medium nonstick skillet over medium-high heat and fry cakes 3–4 minutes per side or until outsides are brown and crispy.

### PER SERVING (1 CAKE)
Calories: 137.56 | Fat: 7.44g | Protein: 16.47g | Sodium: 293mg | Fiber: 0.029g | Carbohydrates: 0.362g | Sugar: 0.181g

# Coconut Shrimp

*This low-fat version of a traditionally fried, tropical dish is easy to prepare and goes well with a fresh salad or pasta dish.*

## Serves 4

¼ cup cornstarch
1 tablespoon Caribbean jerk
  seasoning
2 large egg whites
1 cup sweetened flaked coconut

1 cup panko bread crumbs
1 teaspoon paprika
1½ pounds large shrimp, peeled and
  deveined

1. Preheat oven to 425°F.
2. Set up three shallow bowls. Place cornstarch and jerk seasoning in the first; egg whites in the second; and coconut, panko, and paprika in the third.
3. Dredge shrimp in the cornstarch mix, then egg whites, then panko mixture, coating shrimp on all sides.
4. Place shrimp on a wire baking rack on a baking sheet to catch any drippings.
5. Bake 10–12 minutes, turning halfway through. Remove and serve warm.

**PER SERVING**
Calories: 218.14 | Fat: 3.01g | Protein: 36.025g | Sodium: 276mg |
Fiber: 0.287g | Carbohydrates: 9.27g | Sugar: 0.177g

# Grilled Tuna Teriyaki

*Tuna steaks are easy to find at most stores and provide a healthy dose of protein and omega-3 fatty acids, much like salmon. This light and fresh-tasting recipe is best enjoyed soon after preparing, but it will last for a few days in the refrigerator, if necessary.*

## Serves 4

2 tablespoons soy sauce
1 tablespoon rice wine
1 tablespoon minced gingerroot

1 clove garlic, minced
4 (6-ounce) tuna steaks
1 tablespoon vegetable oil

1. Add soy sauce, rice wine, ginger, and garlic together in a bowl or resealable bag, stirring well. Add tuna to the marinade, turning to coat, and then marinate in the refrigerator at least 30 minutes.
2. When ready to cook, preheat a grill to medium heat, lightly coating with vegetable oil.
3. Transfer fish to grill and discard marinade. Cook tuna 3–6 minutes per side or until fully cooked through.

**PER SERVING**
Calories: 283.44 | Fat: 11.66g | Protein: 39.7g | Sodium: 331mg | Fiber: 0.11g | Carbohydrates: 1.37g | Sugar: 0.168g

# Southwestern Fajitas

*Fajitas are a very flexible meal. Once cooked and prepared, they can be reheated and eaten alone or served with tortillas and rice for extra carbs. You can also serve these with shredded Mexican cheese and low-fat sour cream.*

## Serves 2

6 ounces boneless, skinless chicken breast, cut into strips

1 teaspoon red pepper flakes

1 teaspoon fajita or taco seasoning

1 (12-ounce) bag mixed fajita vegetables

1. Season chicken with red pepper flakes and fajita seasoning. Add to a medium nonstick skillet over medium-high heat and cook 8–10 minutes. Once cooked, remove and set aside.
2. Cook vegetables in pan and mix in chicken once vegetables are fully cooked, about 4–6 minutes.

**PER SERVING**

Calories: 100 | Fat: 2g | Protein: 18g | Sodium: 195mg | Fiber: 0g | Carbohydrates: 0g | Sugar: 0g

# Lemon-Herb Grilled Chicken Salad

*A fresh take on grilled salad, this dish is very refreshing and perfect for the summer.*

**Serves 1**

4 ounces grilled skinless chicken breast, sliced

1 cup mixed greens

1 tablespoon olive oil

1 tablespoon lemon juice

½ teaspoon garlic salt

¼ teaspoon dried rosemary

Mix all ingredients in a medium bowl and serve cold.

**PER SERVING**

Calories: 251 | Fat: 16g | Protein: 24g | Sodium: 240mg | Fiber: 0g | Carbohydrates: 1g | Sugar: 0g

# Pulled-Chicken BBQ Sandwiches

*A very easy way to serve shredded chicken. You can use any sauce you like, including barbecue, hot wing sauce, ranch, or whatever else your favorite sauce may be.*

**Serves 1**

4 ounces shredded slow-cooked chicken

2 tablespoons barbecue sauce (or any other sauce of your choice)
1 whole-wheat hamburger bun

1. In a medium bowl, mix chicken and sauce until chicken is coated completely. (It's best if chicken is heated.)
2. Place chicken on sandwich bun and serve.

**PER SERVING**

Calories: 316 | Fat: 3g | Protein: 29g | Sodium: 1,003mg | Fiber: 4g | Carbohydrates: 43g | Sugar: 14g

### "Detox" with Lemons

While most detox diets are worthless, as your liver does a fine job cleansing you from the inside out, lemons are very beneficial and help support the detoxification process. Lemons are very alkalizing for your body, which means they help maintain a stable pH balance. They are also very good for the liver, a very important organ in the body, and lemon juice is thought to be very cleansing internally.

# Greek Butterflied Chicken

*This delicious recipe is bursting with flavor. Be sure to purchase regular chicken breasts rather than thin-sliced so they can be cut appropriately.*

### Serves 4

1 pound boneless, skinless chicken breasts
½ cup feta cheese
1 (8-ounce) package sun-dried tomatoes

2 tablespoons pesto
¼ teaspoon salt
½ teaspoon freshly ground black pepper

1. Preheat oven to 350°F.
2. Butterfly chicken breasts by slicing along the side of each breast lengthwise.
3. Lay open breasts and place cheese, tomatoes, and pesto on one side of each, then fold other side of breast over filling mixture, using a toothpick to hold stuffed breasts shut, if necessary.
4. Season with salt and pepper and bake 35–40 minutes or until juices run clear.

**PER SERVING**
Calories: 232 | Fat: 8g | Protein: 29g | Sodium: 144mg | Fiber: 3g | Carbohydrates: 13g | Sugar: 9g

### Get Saucy for Maximum Flavor

Anytime you're eating precooked meat, mix up your flavor game with a variety of sauces. Barbecue sauce, hot sauce, mustard, ranch, blue cheese, ketchup…the options are endless, so there is no excuse to eat dry, boring food.

# Beer Can Chicken

*This classic barbecue recipe uses beer to add a lot of moisture to your chicken from the inside. It'll be dripping with juices when you cut it open. You can also prepare the recipe with a can of Coke if you don't want to use alcohol.*

## Serves 4

1 (3–5-pound) whole medium chicken

2 tablespoons olive oil or other vegetable oil

1 tablespoon salt

1 tablespoon freshly ground black pepper

2 tablespoons chopped fresh thyme leaves or 1 tablespoon dried thyme

1 (12-ounce) can beer, room temperature

1. Prepare grill for indirect heat cooking by turning on only one side of burners to medium-high and allowing entire grill to heat to 350°F.
2. Remove innards from chicken and discard. Brush chicken lightly with oil.
3. In a small bowl, combine salt, pepper, and thyme and cover chicken with rub mixture.
4. Open beer, pour out half, and use a knife to carefully cut openings into the top half of the open can. Carefully stand the chicken upright, so that the can is inside its cavity, and place the entire chicken on the cool side of the grill, making sure it stands up on its own. Cover grill.
5. Do not open the grill for at least 1 hour, then check every 15 minutes until fully cooked. A thermometer inserted should read 160–165°F when fully cooked.
6. Remove, allow to rest at least 10 minutes, then cut and serve.

**PER SERVING**

Calories: 368 | Fat: 14g | Protein: 49g | Sodium: 144mg | Fiber: 1g | Carbohydrates: 4g | Sugar: 0g

# Argentinian-Style Grilled Sirloin

*A delicious twist on a traditional sirloin, this minimalist recipe allows the flavor of the steak to come through while providing a mild kick from the fresh seasonings.*

**Serves 2**

2 tablespoons water
½ cup chopped fresh parsley
½ cup chopped fresh cilantro
1 tablespoon lemon juice
1 tablespoon olive oil

¼ teaspoon salt
¼ teaspoon freshly ground black pepper
½ teaspoon red pepper flakes
2 (4-ounce) sirloin steaks

1. In a medium bowl, combine water, parsley, cilantro, lemon juice, oil, salt, black pepper, and red pepper flakes. Mix well.
2. Place steak on grill rack or skillet over medium-high heat and cook about 4 minutes per side.
3. Transfer steak to cutting board and let stand 10 minutes. Thinly slice steaks across the grain. Top with parsley and cilantro mixture before serving.

**PER SERVING**
Calories: 222 | Fat: 13g | Protein: 24g | Sodium: 365mg | Fiber: 1g | Carbohydrates: 2g | Sugar: 0g

# Steakhouse Blue Cheese Burger

*This delicious burger combines the rich taste of beef with the sharp kick of blue cheese, reminiscent of a blue cheese–crusted filet mignon. Serve on a burger bun or with a fresh side salad.*

## Serves 4

1 pound lean ground beef
1 large egg
¼ cup bread crumbs

1 tablespoon steak seasoning
½ cup blue cheese crumbles

1. In a large bowl, combine beef, egg, bread crumbs, and seasoning. Form mixture into four evenly shaped patties.
2. Start to cook patties over a grill or medium skillet preheated to medium-high heat. Cook for about 3–4 minutes on the first side then flip; sprinkle blue cheese crumbles on top of the patties and allow to melt as it cooks to your desired level of doneness.

**PER SERVING**
Calories: 301 | Fat: 18g | Protein: 28g | Sodium: 376mg | Fiber: 0g | Carbohydrates: 5g | Sugar: 1g

# Hearty Beef Stew

*Prep time is quick for this stew, and you can add everything to the slow cooker before you leave for work, ensuring you'll come home to a tender, fresh dinner.*

## Serves 4

4 medium red potatoes, cut into quarters
⅓ cup flour
½ teaspoon salt
¼ teaspoon freshly ground black pepper

1 pound beef stew meat
1 (14-ounce) can diced tomatoes, with liquid
2 cups water
3 cups frozen stir-fry vegetables

1. Add potatoes, flour, salt, pepper, beef, tomatoes, and water to slow cooker and mix well.
2. Cook on low 7–8 hours, until beef and potatoes are tender.
3. Add frozen stir-fry vegetables, cook another 30 minutes, and serve.

**PER SERVING**

Calories: 281 | Fat: 8g | Protein: 27g | Sodium: 362mg | Fiber: 3g | Carbohydrates: 24g | Sugar: 3g

# Swedish-Style Meatballs

*These homemade meatballs are much healthier than the frozen meatballs you can buy at the store. To serve in traditional Swedish fashion, serve with gravy and lingonberry jam.*

## Makes 20 meatballs

1 teaspoon olive oil
1 small onion, peeled and minced
1 clove garlic, minced
1 stalk celery, minced
¼ cup minced fresh parsley
1 pound lean ground beef
1 large egg

¼ cup bread crumbs
½ teaspoon salt
¼ teaspoon freshly ground black pepper
½ teaspoon allspice
2 cups beef stock

1. Heat oil in a large skillet over medium heat and sauté onions and garlic 5 minutes.
2. Add celery and parsley and cook 3 more minutes or until celery softens, then set aside.
3. In a large bowl, combine beef, egg, onion mixture, bread crumbs, salt, pepper, and allspice, mixing well. Form into roughly twenty balls, using about 2 tablespoons of meat mixture for each.
4. Add beef stock to the pan that the celery cooked in and bring to a boil. Add meatballs, cover, and cook 20 minutes, stirring occasionally.
5. Serve warm.

**PER SERVING (1 MEATBALL)**
Calories: 56 | Fat: 3g | Protein: 6g | Sodium: 79mg | Fiber: 0g | Carbohydrates: 2g | Sugar: 3g

# Beef and Broccoli Kebabs

*These kebabs are full of healthy fats and nutrients from the broccoli and are quick and easy to throw on the grill for those summer parties.*

**Serves 4**

⅓ cup soy sauce

¼ cup brown sugar substitute

2 tablespoons lime juice

1 tablespoon ground ginger

1 pound lean sirloin steak, cut into cubes

2 cups whole broccoli florets

2 tablespoons olive oil

3 tablespoons freshly ground black pepper

1. In a large bowl, mix soy sauce, sugar substitute, lime juice, and ginger. Add steak and toss until coated. Cover bowl and marinate in the refrigerator at least 30 minutes.
2. When ready to cook, toss broccoli in oil, remove steak from marinade, and place meat and vegetables on eight metal grilling skewers. Season with pepper.
3. Grill over medium-high heat until cooked to desired doneness, about 6–8 minutes for medium-rare, longer if you want a higher cook temperature, and serve.

**PER SERVING**
Calories: 256 | Fat: 13g | Protein: 27g | Sodium: 791mg | Fiber: 3g | Carbohydrates: 9g | Sugar: 1g

## Clean Your Equipment

Food safety is a crucial part of staying healthy, and a big part of this is keeping your grill clean between uses. Just because you're cooking over a hot fire doesn't mean you're necessarily killing any bacteria left on the grill. To keep your food safe, thoroughly brush your grill grates clean with a grill cleaning brush after each use.

# Orange-Flavored Beef Stir-Fry

*This low-fat spin on a classic Chinese dish is a healthy alternative that's easy to prepare at home. This is a mild recipe; for extra spice, try adding some hot sauce or chili peppers.*

## Serves 4

2 medium oranges, whole; plus
  2 medium oranges, peeled and
  sliced; divided
2 cloves garlic, minced
2 tablespoons soy sauce

1 tablespoon cornstarch
1 tablespoon cold water
1½ pounds sirloin, cut into thin strips
3 green onions, sliced
1 tablespoon sesame seeds

1. In a small bowl, grate zest from 1 orange and squeeze juice from 2 oranges. Add garlic and soy sauce, and stir.
2. In a separate small bowl, mix cornstarch with cold water and add to orange juice bowl.
3. In a large skillet over medium heat, cook beef strips until browned on all sides and cooked to desired doneness, roughly 6–8 minutes.
4. Set beef aside and pour juice mix into skillet, boiling until juice thickens. Return beef to skillet and add orange slices, green onion, and sesame seeds, tossing well before serving.

**PER SERVING**

Calories: 373 | Fat: 13g | Protein: 38g | Sodium: 365mg | Fiber: 5g | Carbohydrates: 25g | Sugar: 17g

## Save Time with Stir-Fry Mixes

If you enjoy making stir-fry dishes, check your frozen vegetable section for premade stir-fry mixes. You can often find frozen packages of assorted vegetables that are ready to throw in the pan with your protein of choice for a quick and healthy meal.

# Quick Ramen with Shredded Chicken

*This recipe is very quick to put together and a good way to use premade chicken. All you need is chicken, a package of ramen, and a few side ingredients to make this delicious dish.*

**Serves 4**

3 cups water

1 (3-ounce) package chicken-flavored ramen noodles, with seasoning package

2 cups cooked, shredded skinless chicken breast

2 bok choy leaves, sliced into strips

1 medium carrot, peeled and sliced

1 teaspoon sesame oil

1. Bring water to a boil in a large pot.
2. Add all other ingredients and simmer 3–5 minutes before serving.

**PER SERVING**
Calories: 225 | Fat: 7g | Protein: 24g | Sodium: 476mg | Fiber: 1g | Carbohydrates: 14g | Sugar: 1g

### Ramen: The Cheapest Carbohydrate
Ramen may take you back to your college days, and yes, it's processed and full of sodium. However, when on a budget, ramen is very cheap, easy to prepare, and comes in all sorts of flavors. If you make it fit your macros, it's perfectly fine to enjoy some cheap ramen from time to time.

# Spicy Buffalo Macaroni and Cheese

*This recipe combines two classic American flavors—buffalo chicken and macaroni and cheese. It contains significantly less fat than you'd get at restaurants that serve mac and cheese, so you can enjoy this dish guilt-free.*

**Serves 2**

2 cups macaroni
1 tablespoon butter
½ cup fat-free shredded Cheddar cheese
6 ounces grilled skinless chicken, cut into strips

2 tablespoons Frank's RedHot Original Cayenne Pepper Sauce
½ cup blue cheese crumbles

1. Cook pasta according to package directions, drain, and return to pot.
2. Stir in butter and Cheddar cheese until cheese begins to melt.
3. Top with grilled chicken, drizzle with hot sauce, add blue cheese, and serve.

**PER SERVING**

Calories: 750 | Fat: 25g | Protein: 48g | Sodium: 612mg | Fiber: 4g | Carbohydrates: 81g | Sugar: 3g

# Traditional Shrimp Scampi

*Shrimp scampi is a delicious meal that is made using simple ingredients. This recipe uses orzo, but you can substitute your favorite pasta, if desired, or serve plain over steamed vegetables to reduce the carbohydrate count in this recipe.*

## Serves 4

1 cup dry orzo
½ teaspoon salt
2 tablespoons chopped fresh parsley
4 tablespoons butter, divided

1½ pounds jumbo shrimp, peeled
   and deveined
1 clove garlic, minced

1. Cook orzo according to package directions. Stir in salt and parsley and set aside.
2. In a medium skillet, heat 2 tablespoons butter over medium-high heat. Sauté shrimp 2–3 minutes or until nearly cooked through and then set aside.
3. Combine remaining 2 tablespoons butter and garlic in pan and cook 30 seconds before returning shrimp to the pan.
4. Mix shrimp and garlic butter well and serve with orzo.

**PER SERVING**
Calories: 249 | Fat: 13g | Protein: 12g | Sodium: 614mg | Fiber: 1g | Carbohydrates: 22g | Sugar: 1g

# Chicken and Pesto Farfalle

*This is a low-fat and high-protein dish with minimal ingredients for an easy preparation.*

## Serves 2

8 ounces dry farfalle
½ cup reserved pasta water
½ pound fresh green beans, ends
  trimmed

½ cup reduced-fat pesto sauce
2 cups grilled skinless chicken, cut
  into bite-sized pieces

1. Cook pasta according to package directions and drain, reserving ½ cup pasta water.
2. Place green beans in a shallow 8" pan with enough fresh water to cover them. Steam beans over medium heat 15 minutes and drain.
3. Combine pasta, pesto, reserved water, chicken, and green beans in a large bowl and stir to combine. This dish can be served hot or refrigerated for later and served chilled.

**PER SERVING**
Calories: 792 | Fat: 20g | Protein: 48g | Sodium: 515mg | Fiber: 7g | Carbohydrates: 99g | Sugar: 12g

# Orzo and Shrimp Salad

*This unique spin on a pasta salad uses orzo, shrimp, and Mediterranean flavors.*

**Serves 4**

8 ounces dry orzo
1 pound cooked shrimp, tails removed
1 cup cherry tomatoes, sliced in half
2 ounces reduced-fat feta cheese
¼ cup chopped basil

1 tablespoon olive oil
1 tablespoon lemon juice
1 teaspoon salt
1 teaspoon freshly ground black pepper

1. Cook pasta according to package directions. Drain and rinse under cool water.
2. Combine orzo with shrimp, tomatoes, feta cheese, basil, oil, and lemon juice in a large bowl.
3. Season with salt and pepper, mix well, and serve.

**PER SERVING**
Calories: 420 | Fat: 9g | Protein: 34g | Sodium: 1,733mg | Fiber: 3g | Carbohydrates: 45g | Sugar: 4g

# Salmon and Spinach Fettuccine

*This dish is packed with omega-3 fatty acids from the salmon and healthy nutrients from the spinach.*

## Serves 2

8 ounces dry fettuccine
¼ cup butter
1 cup fat-free milk
1 tablespoon flour or flour substitute
1 cup freshly grated Parmesan cheese

½ pound smoked salmon, chopped
1 cup chopped fresh spinach
2 tablespoons capers
¼ cup chopped sun-dried tomatoes
½ cup chopped fresh oregano

1. Bring a large pot of lightly salted water to a boil. Add fettuccine and cook 11–13 minutes.
2. In a medium saucepan over medium heat, melt butter and stir in milk.
3. Mix in flour to thicken. Gradually stir in Parmesan until melted.
4. Crumble salmon into sauce. Stir in spinach, capers, sun-dried tomatoes, and oregano. Cook and stir about 3 minutes, and serve over fettuccine.

**PER SERVING**
Calories: 1,048 | Fat: 45g | Protein: 61g | Sodium: 1,815mg | Fiber: 5g | Carbohydrates: 99g | Sugar: 12g

# Light Fettuccine Alfredo

*Fettuccine Alfredo is one of the heaviest, fattiest, cream-based pasta dishes around...at least it was, before this low-fat version.*

## Serves 2

12 ounces dry fettuccine

2½ teaspoons salt, divided

1 head broccoli, cut into florets, stalk peeled and sliced

1½ cups skim milk

1 tablespoon unsalted butter

1 tablespoon flour

¾ cup freshly grated Parmesan cheese, plus more for serving

1. Cook pasta according to package directions. Drain.
2. Bring a pot of water with 1 teaspoon salt to a boil and cook broccoli 3 minutes until tender.
3. Heat milk and butter in a large saucepan over low heat and slowly whisk in flour until thickened.
4. Remove from heat and stir in Parmesan and remaining salt. Add pasta and broccoli and cook, stirring over low heat until heated through, about 3–5 minutes.

**PER SERVING**

Calories: 958 | Fat: 21g | Protein: 46g | Sodium: 1,278mg | Fiber: 8g | Carbohydrates: 144g | Sugar: 16g

# Corn and Bacon Chowder

*A filling, higher-fat soup, this recipe is perfect for low-carb days on your plan.*

**Serves 4**

½ cup chopped celery
½ cup chopped onion
2 (16-ounce) packages frozen corn, thawed and divided
2 cups skim milk, divided
½ teaspoon salt

¼ teaspoon freshly ground black pepper
¾ cup fat-free shredded Cheddar cheese
2 slices bacon, cooked and crumbled

1. Sauté celery, onion, and one package corn in a stockpot over medium heat 5 minutes or until tender.
2. In a blender, blend remaining package corn and 1 cup skim milk until smooth.
3. Add blended corn and milk mixture to pan with vegetables. Add remaining milk, salt, pepper, and cheese.
4. Cook, stirring constantly, until cheese melts. Serve topped with crumbled bacon bits.

**PER SERVING**

Calories: 347 | Fat: 9g | Protein: 20g | Sodium: 612mg | Fiber: 7g | Carbohydrates: 56g | Sugar: 28g

### Crumbled Bacon for Maximum Flavor

One way to add amazing flavor to your favorite dishes is by sprinkling on some crumbled bacon bits instead of using traditional salt. You need to be careful, as this does increase the fat content, but it's a lot tastier and a lot more fun than sticking with regular salt. Cook 4–6 slices until crispy, allow to cool, crumble into a resealable plastic bag or airtight container, and store until ready to use.

# Garlic Cheddar Cauliflower Soup

*This is a cheesy, delicious, and healthy soup that's sure to please everyone, even those who don't like cauliflower, as the seasonings provide a nice flavor.*

## Serves 2

2 tablespoons olive oil
1 small yellow onion, peeled and chopped
2 cloves garlic, minced
1 medium cauliflower head, rinsed and chopped
4 cups low-sodium chicken broth
½ cup grated Parmesan cheese

1. Heat oil in a large saucepan over medium heat and add onion and garlic.
2. After 5 minutes, add cauliflower and chicken stock, bringing to a boil.
3. Reduce heat and simmer 20 minutes or until cauliflower is soft.
4. Transfer mixture to a blender and blend in batches until smooth.
5. Return to pan, stir in Parmesan, and heat through before serving.

### PER SERVING

Calories: 341 | Fat: 21g | Protein: 17g | Sodium: 670mg | Fiber: 6g | Carbohydrates: 24g | Sugar: 7g

# Garlic Mashed Sweet Potatoes

*This recipe takes a bit longer to prepare, but the garlic provides a delicious spin on traditional mashed potatoes.*

## Serves 5

4 sweet potatoes, peeled and cubed
1 teaspoon salt
1 tablespoon butter
3 cloves garlic, crushed
½ cup skim milk
2 tablespoons light sour cream

1. Place potatoes in a slow cooker, adding enough water to cover them. Add salt and cook on low 4 hours or until potatoes are soft.
2. In a small saucepan over medium heat, sauté garlic in butter for 3 minutes or until garlic is slightly browned, and then stir in milk and sour cream, mixing well.
3. Drain potatoes and return to slow cooker, adding sauce. Mash with a potato masher or with a blender until smooth.

**PER SERVING**
Calories: 131 | Fat: 3g | Protein: 3g | Sodium: 539mg | Fiber: 3g | Carbohydrates: 23g | Sugar: 6g

### Boost Your Health with Garlic

In addition to being very tasty, garlic packs a lot of nutrients and is very good for boosting your immune system. If you find yourself coming down with a cold or feeling a bit under the weather for any other reason, try some garlic. You can supplement with garlic capsules but adding it to your food is the easiest method, and it'll make just about anything taste better.

# Cabbage Slaw

*This low-calorie side is packed with healthy nutrients and fiber to keep you full and healthy.*

## Serves 4

½ small head cabbage, shredded
½ medium red bell pepper, seeded and sliced
¼ small red onion, peeled and sliced

2 tablespoons olive oil
5 teaspoons apple cider vinegar
¼ teaspoon salt

Toss all ingredients in a large bowl until mixed well and allow to chill at least 15 minutes in the refrigerator before serving.

**PER SERVING**

Calories: 96 | Fat: 7g | Protein: 2g | Sodium: 167mg | Fiber: 3g | Carbohydrates: 8g | Sugar: 5g

### Moisten Your Cabbage with Salt

While shredded, fresh cabbage seems very dry and bland, it actually has a very high moisture content. Salt pulls water from things, so when you mix salt into your cabbage and let it sit for a while, you'll notice all sorts of juices coming out of the cabbage. Using salt is an easy, zero-calorie way to add some flavor and moisture to your cabbage dishes.

# Garlic Parmesan Fries

*This recipe makes enough to serve two people, but you can prepare it in bulk to have on hand for the rest of the week or to feed a large party.*

## Serves 2

1 teaspoon olive oil
1 clove garlic, crushed
1 large potato, peeled and cut into fries

½ teaspoon salt
1 tablespoon grated Parmesan cheese
1 tablespoon chopped fresh parsley

1. Preheat oven to 425°F.
2. In a medium bowl, combine oil and garlic and toss potatoes in mixture, coating well.
3. Arrange fries on a baking sheet, spreading evenly, and top with salt. Bake 10 minutes per side.
4. Remove, top with Parmesan and parsley, and serve.

**PER SERVING**
Calories: 163 | Fat: 3g | Protein: 4g | Sodium: 669mg | Fiber: 5g | Carbohydrates: 30g | Sugar: 2g

### Bake Your Way to Better Health

French fries are traditionally, well, fried. The frying process can add trans fats and omega-6 fatty acids, which can cause inflammation and should be avoided. When you slice your fresh potatoes up and crisp them in the oven instead, you have a healthy side dish that's still delicious. Try mixing up your seasonings for variety— spicy seasonings, garlic salt, and ranch seasonings all work very well with home-made French fries.

# Cilantro Lime Low-Carb Rice

*Using riced cauliflower is a great substitute for traditional rice recipes when you need to lower your daily carb intake.*

## Serves 4

1 (10-ounce) bag riced cauliflower (thawed or fresh)
3 tablespoons water

1 medium lime, juiced and zested
½ cup chopped fresh cilantro

1. Combine riced cauliflower and water in a large microwave-safe bowl and microwave 3–5 minutes or until cauliflower is soft.
2. Remove and add lime juice, zest, and cilantro to bowl. Mix well before serving.

**PER SERVING**
Calories: 176 | Fat: 2g | Protein: 14g | Sodium: 170mg | Fiber: 17g | Carbohydrates: 35g | Sugar: 16g

### Low-Carb Rice at Home
Cauliflower is fairly neutral in flavor, particularly when you add other flavors and seasonings to it. If you're unable to find riced cauliflower at your local store, it's quite easy to make at home. Simply take a head of cauliflower, chop it up into bits, and run it through the food processor until well-chopped. You can steam up these little bits as a low-carb rice substitute.

# Buffalo and Blue Cheese Brussels Sprouts

*If you want a meat-free and low-fat version of buffalo wings for the big game, these Brussels sprouts are a healthy alternative to fried wings.*

## Serves 4

2 tablespoons olive oil
1 pound Brussels sprouts, trimmed
  and halved

¼ cup Frank's RedHot Original
  Cayenne Pepper Sauce
2 tablespoons blue cheese crumbles

1. Preheat oven to 425°F.
2. While oven heats, sauté Brussels sprouts in oil in a large skillet over medium heat about 5 minutes until softened.
3. Spread on a baking sheet and roast in the oven an additional 10–12 minutes.
4. Transfer to a large bowl, toss with hot sauce until well coated, and top with blue cheese crumbles before serving.

**PER SERVING**

Calories: 123 | Fat: 8g | Protein: 5g | Sodium: 639mg | Fiber: 4g | Carbohydrates: 10g | Sugar: 3g

### Fire Up Your Metabolism with Hot Sauce

Hot sauce contains capsaicin, which may slightly increase your metabolism. Adding hot sauce to your meals won't be enough to make you lose a lot of weight, but it certainly can't hurt anything, and it makes your food taste better. If you're low on calories and want to keep your metabolism up, eating spicy foods may be just what you need.

1.

# Cinnamon-Apple Protein Bars

*If you rely on protein bars as healthy snacks, you'll love this healthy, homemade recipe. Say goodbye to stomach cramps from weird protein bar ingredients, and say hello to your new healthy recipe.*

## Serves 4

¾ cup dry oats
¼ cup oat bran
6 large egg whites
1 (30-gram) scoop vanilla protein powder

2 tablespoons unsweetened apple-sauce
¼ teaspoon baking powder
1 (1-gram) packet stevia
1 teaspoon cinnamon
2 tablespoons olive oil
2 medium apples, peeled and diced

1. Preheat oven to 350°F.
2. Combine all ingredients except apples in blender until well mixed.
3. Pour into a large bowl, add apples, and mix well.
4. Spread mixture in a 10" × 13" lightly greased glass baking dish and bake 30 minutes.
5. Cut into four equal squares and allow to cool.

**PER SERVING**
Calories: 170 | Fat: 2g | Protein: 15g | Sodium: 43mg | Fiber: 4g | Carbohydrates: 27g | Sugar: 10g

### Save Your Gut with Homemade Bars

To save calories, many popular protein bars on the market use various sugar alcohols and other additives to add flavor without using actual sugar. It's very common for these ingredients to cause digestive pain and cramping. If you've ever eaten a protein bar and noticed discomfort, there's a good chance it was the sugar alcohols, not the protein itself.

# Easy Kale Chips

*Kale is the healthiest green on the planet, but it can be quite bitter to eat raw. Making kale chips is super easy and results in an addicting and healthy snack.*

## Serves 2

2 cups raw kale leaves, washed and torn into smaller pieces

1 tablespoon olive oil

2 teaspoons garlic salt

1 tablespoon grated Parmesan cheese

1. Preheat oven to 400°F.
2. Dry kale thoroughly using paper towels or a salad spinner; mix it with oil in a large bowl, coating each piece well.
3. Spread kale out evenly over a baking sheet covered with aluminum foil.
4. Sprinkle with garlic salt and Parmesan.
5. Bake 8–12 minutes or until it reaches your desired crispness.

**PER SERVING**

Calories: 81 | Fat: 8g | Protein: 2g | Sodium: 2,023mg | Fiber: 1g | Carbohydrates: 2g | Sugar: 0g

# Shamrock Shake Protein Smoothie

*This cold, minty, refreshing protein smoothie tastes like a milkshake—a healthy one.*

## Serves 1

1 (30-gram) scoop chocolate protein powder

1 teaspoon mint extract

½ cup skim milk

1 cup cold water

1 teaspoon cocoa powder

1 (1-gram) packet stevia

5 ice cubes

Place all ingredients in a blender and blend until smooth. Serve immediately.

**PER SERVING**

Calories: 180 | Fat: 2g | Protein: 31g | Sodium: 104mg | Fiber: 1g | Carbohydrates: 9g | Sugar: 8g

# Kefir and Chia Super Pudding

*Kefir is loaded with probiotics and good bacteria. When combined with chia seeds, a superfood, it makes for a very healthy snack.*

**Serves 2**

1 cup plain kefir
1 cup mixed berries

3 tablespoons chia seeds
½ cup unsweetened almond milk

1. Place kefir and berries in a blender and blend until smooth.
2. Pour mixture into a large bowl and stir in chia seeds and almond milk. Allow to set in the refrigerator at least 6 hours before serving.

**PER SERVING**

Calories: 205 | Fat: 8g | Protein: 10g | Sodium: 109mg | Fiber: 9g | Carbohydrates: 26g | Sugar: 13g

### What Is Kefir, Anyway?

Many believe that kefir is similar to quality yogurts because it contains healthy probiotics that are good for your gut. This is true, but there's more to the story. Kefir also contains yeast and the types of good bacteria that can actually remain in your gut and help you maintain a healthy digestive environment. In contrast, regular yogurt just passes through without providing many benefits.

# Homemade Tortilla Chips

*Everyone loves chips and salsa, and this quick and easy homemade recipe gives you peace of mind about what you're eating.*

## Serves 6

10 medium corn tortillas
3 tablespoons lime juice

1 tablespoon olive oil
1 teaspoon salt

1. Preheat oven to 350°F.
2. Cut tortillas into chip-sized pieces and spread evenly on a lightly oiled baking sheet.
3. Mix lime juice and oil in a small bowl and brush or spray on tortillas, then lightly salt tortillas.
4. Cook 12–14 minutes or until crispy, turning halfway through.

**PER SERVING**

Calories: 109 | Fat: 3g | Protein: 2g | Sodium: 407mg | Fiber: 3g | Carbohydrates: 18g | Sugar: 1g

# Protein Fluff

*This delicious treat is very filling and will keep you feeling satisfied and energized. Use any combinations of protein and berries that you prefer. Whey protein will work in this recipe but won't "fluff" as well as the casein.*

## Serves 2

½ cup frozen berries, slightly thawed
2 (30-gram) scoops chocolate casein protein
¼ cup skim milk
1 (1-gram) packet stevia or your sweetener of choice

1. Add all ingredients in a medium bowl and stir. The mixture should have a thick, pudding-like texture. (You can eat it now as is or continue to next step to make it fluffy.)
2. Using a power blender, blend mixture on medium 5–10 minutes until it fluffs up.

**PER SERVING**
Calories: 116 | Fat: 1g | Protein: 20g | Sodium: 64mg | Fiber: 1g | Carbohydrates: 8g | Sugar: 5g

### How to Make Protein Fluff Even Fluffier

By mixing all the ingredients in a bowl, you already have a satisfying, filling treat. If you have a blender available, however, mixing it for 5–10 minutes can double or even triple the volume, making this taste like fruity whipped cream. You may actually find it hard to avoid eating the entire bowl, so it's a great way to fill your stomach with very few calories.

# Triple-Berry Yogurt Parfait

*This is a fun and sweet treat that's perfect for a relaxing day. You can choose high- or low-fat ingredients to make this fit your caloric goals.*

## Serves 2

1 cup vanilla Greek yogurt
½ cup fresh blueberries
½ cup fresh blackberries

½ cup fresh raspberries
½ cup fat-free whipped cream
½ cup granola or high-fiber cereal

In a glass or small bowl, layer the ingredients in a visually pleasing manner or mix it all up to enjoy.

**PER SERVING**

Calories: 238 | Fat: 5g | Protein: 15g | Sodium: 56mg | Fiber: 7g |
Carbohydrates: 38g | Sugar: 23g

### Berries: Micronutrient Bombs

Berries are very rich in vitamins, minerals, and antioxidants that help your body flush out all the bad free radicals produced by stress. They are also high in fiber and support healthy digestion. In addition, their natural sugars help satisfy your sweet tooth.

# Frozen Chocolate Bananas

*The perfect summer treat, quick to prepare and easy to grab and enjoy.*

**Serves 2**

2 medium bananas
4 ounces dark chocolate

½ cup ground peanuts, or any topping you prefer

1. Peel bananas, cut in half, and place in freezer until firm.
2. Melt dark chocolate in a bowl in the microwave 3–5 minutes or until soft, or over the stove until soft.
3. Remove bananas from freezer and roll them in melted chocolate to cover, sprinkle with nuts or topping of choice, and return to the freezer until ready to enjoy.

**PER SERVING**

Calories: 580 | Fat: 35g | Protein: 13g | Sodium: 13mg | Fiber: 9g | Carbohydrates: 68g | Sugar: 46g

### Bananas for Exercise

When you are very active, especially during the summer months, it's very important to stay hydrated, as you can sweat out electrolytes. Bananas are not only a great source of natural sugar, they are full of potassium to keep you hydrated and help prevent cramping.

# Peanut Butter Protein Cookies

*The protein and fat in this recipe will keep you full with minimal carbohydrates. It's perfect for your sweet tooth on those low-carb days.*

## Makes 10 cookies

1 cup natural peanut butter
2 large egg whites
1 (30-gram) scoop vanilla protein powder

¾ cup stevia
1 teaspoon cinnamon

1. Preheat oven to 350°F.
2. Place all ingredients into a medium bowl and stir.
3. Shape dough into round cookies and spread out on a greased baking sheet, leaving 1" between cookies.
4. Bake 10 minutes, cool, and serve.

**PER SERVING (1 COOKIE)**

Calories: 168 | Fat: 13g | Protein: 8g | Sodium: 95mg | Fiber: 2g | Carbohydrates: 8g | Sugar: 3g

## Cycle Your Nut Sources

Nuts are one of the best natural sources of fat available and even contain a little bit of protein. If you get tired of regular peanut butter, try cycling your nut butters. Almond butter, cashew butter, and even sunflower seed butter are all delicious and healthy options you can use for variety.

# Protein Cheesecake

*Cheesecake is notorious for being a high-fat recipe, but this version is incredibly low in fat with a high protein content and delicious flavor. Top with berries for an extrasweet nutritional treat.*

## Makes 1 cheesecake (Serves 12)

24 ounces fat-free cream cheese
2 (30-gram) scoops vanilla whey
　protein
¾ cup stevia

1 teaspoon vanilla extract
3 large eggs
1 tablespoon lemon juice

1. Preheat oven to 350°F.
2. Place ingredients in a large bowl and mix with a hand mixer on medium speed.
3. Pour mixture into a 9" pie pan coated with nonstick cooking spray.
4. Bake 45 minutes and refrigerate 3 hours or until ready to serve.

**PER SERVING**
Calories: 177 | Fat: 3g | Protein: 24g | Sodium: 800mg | Fiber: 0g |
Carbohydrates: 11g | Sugar: 7g

## Use Flavored Proteins in Your Baking

Most recipes can be made with chocolate or vanilla protein powders, which are readily available just about anywhere and are generally mild-flavored and safe to use. If you're feeling a little adventurous, head to your local supplement shop and check out their selection. You can often find many more flavors than you'd find at your grocery store if you want to move beyond chocolate and vanilla.

# Peanut Butter Banana Frozen Greek Yogurt

*This super quick, super delicious treat is perfect for satisfying your sweet tooth with natural ingredients. If you want to experiment with flavors, take out the protein and add lemon juice for a tart treat, or frozen berries.*

## Serves 1

½ cup Greek yogurt

1 medium frozen banana, sliced

2 tablespoons natural peanut butter

Blend all ingredients in a blender or food processor until smooth and serve immediately.

**PER SERVING**

Calories: 362 | Fat: 16g | Protein: 20g | Sodium: 139mg | Fiber: 5g | Carbohydrates: 41g | Sugar: 23g

# Three-Ingredient Cinnamon Pecan Bites

*Minimal ingredients provide a great source of healthy fats for sustained energy, and the end result is delicious and easy to prepare.*

## Makes 10–12 cookies

10 pitted dates, soaked in water 15 minutes

2 cups raw pecans

2 teaspoons cinnamon

1. Preheat oven to 350°F.
2. Drain dates and combine all ingredients in food processor, blending until smooth.
3. Shape into small balls and place on lined baking sheets 1" apart.
4. Bake 10–12 minutes and allow to cool before serving.

**PER SERVING (1 COOKIE)**

Calories: 228 | Fat: 16g | Protein: 3g | Sodium: 0mg | Fiber: 4g | Carbohydrates: 22g | Sugar: 17g

### Bake with Dates

Dates may not be a popular snack, but these sticky-sweet treats make a great natural sweetener for your baking needs. In addition to adding natural sugars, dates can add moisture and fiber, giving your recipes extra richness and flavor without the need for sugar and butter.

# Appendix: Macro-Rich Foods

## Carbohydrates

- Acai berries
- Apples
- Bananas
- Beans
- Beets
- Black-eyed peas
- Blackberries
- Blueberries
- Buckwheat
- Bulgur
- Cantaloupe
- Chickpeas
- Chips
- Corn
- Couscous
- Dates
- Energy bars
- Farro
- Grapefruit
- Grapes
- Green peas
- Lentils
- Lima beans
- Mango
- Millet
- Muffins
- Multigrain hot cereal
- Oatmeal
- Oranges
- Pancakes
- Parsnips
- Pasta
- Peaches
- Pears
- Pineapple
- Plums
- Potatoes
- Pretzels
- Pumpkin
- Quinoa
- Raisins
- Rice
- Sourdough bread
- Squash
- Strawberries
- Sweet potatoes
- Waffles
- Watermelon
- Whole-wheat bread
- Yams

## Fat-Rich Foods

- Almonds
- Avocado
- Bacon
- Beef
- Butter
- Canola oil
- Cashews
- Chia seeds
- Cocoa butter
- Coconut
- Coconut oil
- Dark chocolate
- Duck
- Edamame
- Egg yolks
- Flaxseed
- Greek yogurt
- Heavy cream
- Hemp seed oil
- Macadamia nuts
- Mackerel
- Olive oil
- Olives
- Parmesan cheese

- Peanut butter
- Peanut oil
- Peanuts
- Pecans
- Pine nuts
- Pistachios
- Salmon
- Sardines
- Sour cream
- Soybeans
- Spirulina
- Sunflower seeds
- Tofu
- Tuna
- Walnuts
- Whole milk

## Protein-Rich Foods

- 2% milk
- Amaranth
- Anchovies
- Asparagus
- Beef
- Bone broth
- Broccoli
- Brussels sprouts

- Canned tuna
- Chicken
- Chorizo
- Cod
- Cottage cheese
- Eggs
- Grapefruit
- Greek yogurt
- Green beans
- Guava
- Halibut
- Hummus
- Kefir
- Kidney beans
- Lentils
- Mushrooms
- Nuts
- Passion fruit
- Pistachios
- Pomegranate
- Pork
- Pumpkin seeds
- Quinoa
- Rainbow trout
- Salmon
- Seitan
- Shrimp

- Soba noodles
- Soybeans
- Squash
- Spinach
- Spirulina
- Sun-dried tomatoes
- Swiss cheese
- Tempeh
- Tilapia
- Tofu
- Tuna
- Turkey
- Unsweetened cocoa powder
- Wheatgrass powder
- Whey protein

# US/Metric Conversion Chart

| VOLUME CONVERSIONS | |
|---|---|
| US Volume Measure | Metric Equivalent |
| ⅛ teaspoon | 0.5 milliliter |
| ¼ teaspoon | 1 milliliter |
| ½ teaspoon | 2 milliliters |
| 1 teaspoon | 5 milliliters |
| ½ tablespoon | 7 milliliters |
| 1 tablespoon (3 teaspoons) | 15 milliliters |
| 2 tablespoons (1 fluid ounce) | 30 milliliters |
| ¼ cup (4 tablespoons) | 60 milliliters |
| ⅓ cup | 90 milliliters |
| ½ cup (4 fluid ounces) | 125 milliliters |
| ⅔ cup | 160 milliliters |
| ¾ cup (6 fluid ounces) | 180 milliliters |
| 1 cup (16 tablespoons) | 250 milliliters |
| 1 pint (2 cups) | 500 milliliters |
| 1 quart (4 cups) | 1 liter (about) |
| WEIGHT CONVERSIONS | |
| US Weight Measure | Metric Equivalent |
| ½ ounce | 15 grams |
| 1 ounce | 30 grams |
| 2 ounces | 60 grams |
| 3 ounces | 85 grams |
| ¼ pound (4 ounces) | 115 grams |
| ½ pound (8 ounces) | 225 grams |
| ¾ pound (12 ounces) | 340 grams |
| 1 pound (16 ounces) | 454 grams |

## OVEN TEMPERATURE CONVERSIONS

| Degrees Fahrenheit | Degrees Celsius |
|---|---|
| 200 degrees F | 95 degrees C |
| 250 degrees F | 120 degrees C |
| 275 degrees F | 135 degrees C |
| 300 degrees F | 150 degrees C |
| 325 degrees F | 160 degrees C |
| 350 degrees F | 180 degrees C |
| 375 degrees F | 190 degrees C |
| 400 degrees F | 205 degrees C |
| 425 degrees F | 220 degrees C |
| 450 degrees F | 230 degrees C |

## BAKING PAN SIZES

| American | Metric |
|---|---|
| 8 × 1½ inch round baking pan | 20 × 4 cm cake tin |
| 9 × 1½ inch round baking pan | 23 × 3.5 cm cake tin |
| 11 × 7 × 1½ inch baking pan | 28 × 18 × 4 cm baking tin |
| 13 × 9 × 2 inch baking pan | 30 × 20 × 5 cm baking tin |
| 2 quart rectangular baking dish | 30 × 20 × 3 cm baking tin |
| 15 × 10 × 2 inch baking pan | 30 × 25 × 2 cm baking tin (Swiss roll tin) |
| 9 inch pie plate | 22 × 4 or 23 × 4 cm pie plate |
| 7 or 8 inch springform pan | 18 or 20 cm springform or loose bottom cake tin |
| 9 × 5 × 3 inch loaf pan | 23 × 13 × 7 cm or 2 lb narrow loaf or pâté tin |
| 1½ quart casserole | 1.5 liter casserole |
| 2 quart casserole | 2 liter casserole |

# Index

## About the Author

Matt Dustin, CSCS, is a personal trainer, author, and online fitness coach based out of San Diego. In addition to earning his bachelor's degree in exercise science, Matt is a certified strength and conditioning specialist and precision nutrition coach. He's been training clients since 2011 and has worked with high-level athletes, models, actors, CEOs, and everyone in between. Matt is the author of *The Everything® Guide to the Carb Cycling Diet* and *The Everything® Guide to Macronutrients*, and he's been featured on AskMen.com, T-Nation.com, Bodybuilding.com, and MuscleandStrength.com, as well as in *Sports Illustrated*, among other outlets.

# Learn the basics
## of the VEGAN DIET!

# VEGAN
# BASICS

### INCLUDES 50+ RECIPES

**Your Guide to the Essentials of a Plant-Based Diet—and How It Can Work for You!**

**VEGAN GUIDELINES**

**STARTER RECIPES**

**LIFESTYLE ADJUSTMENTS**

## Pick Up or Download Your Copy Today!

adamsmedia
An Imprint of Simon & Schuster
A CBS COMPANY